We're all learning that sitting too much is dangerous—but who knew that standing up doesn't fix the problem? *Don't Just Sit There* offers a true alternative to our sedentary workplaces, giving concrete steps to becoming more healthy and more productive.
—Robb Wolf, *New York Times* bestselling author of *The Paleo Solution*

The next time you are told to "take a seat," you may reconsider how you configure yourself. Katy's text rearranges the physiological blind spots caused by the negative consequences of body idleness. Katy's book captures your attention from eyeball to footfall.
—Jill Miller, author of *The Roll Model: A Step by Step Guide to Erase Pain, Improve Mobility and Live Better in your Body*

As someone who was gung-ho about my standing desk until it started making me ache all day, I had a light-bulb moment while reading this book. It's not the desks; it's our whole techno-bound lifestyle. But this book isn't just a literal eye-opener (my work space is ruining my eyes, too?), it also provides myriad actionable items to improve all aspects of your health. This book is a great how-to manual for examining and creating better movement and a better quality of life.
—Becca Borawski Jenkins, Managing Editor, *Breaking Muscle*

Katy Bowman's *Don't Just Sit There* is more than just timely, it is absolutely necessary in our increasingly technological lives. She offers sane, scientifically validated, and approachable techniques for getting the most out of our bodies, even when we do find ourselves sitting. What's more, she tempers the sitting sensationalism, taking us past the memes and headlines, empowering us with the knowledge and tools we need to care for our frames for a lifetime.
—Daniel Vitalis, health motivator, author, *ReWild Yourself Magazine*

# DON'T
## JUST *SIT*
# THERE

**TRANSITIONING TO A STANDING AND DYNAMIC WORKSTATION FOR WHOLE-BODY HEALTH**

# DON'T
## JUST *SIT*
## THERE

**TRANSITIONING TO A STANDING AND DYNAMIC
WORKSTATION FOR WHOLE-BODY HEALTH**

# KATY BOWMAN, M.S.

**FOREWORD BY MARK SISSON**

PROPRIOMETRICS
PRESS

Printed in the United States of America.
First Printing, 2015 ISBN-13: 978-1-943370-00-9
Library of Congress Control Number: 2015946726
Propriometrics Press: propriometricspress.com
Cover Design: Zsofi Koller, zsofikoller.com
Interior Design: Agnes Koller, figdesign.ca
Illustrations: Jillian Nicol
Cover image: iStock.com/OJO Images
Photographs: Michael Curran, Galina Denzel
Author photograph: J. Jurgensen Photography

The information in this book should not be used for diagnosis or treatment, or as a substitute for professional medical care. Please consult with your health care provider prior to attempting any treatment on yourself or another individual.

Publisher's Cataloging-In-Publication Data
(Prepared by The Donohue Group, Inc.)

Bowman, Katy.
    Don't just sit there : transitioning to a standing and dynamic workstation for whole-body health / Katy Bowman, M.S. ; foreword by Mark Sisson ; illustrations: Jillian Nicol.

    pages : illustrations ; cm

    Includes bibliographical references and index.
    ISBN: 978-1-943370-00-9

    1. Exercise therapy. 2. Sedentary behavior--Physiological effect. 3. Human loco-motion--Health aspects. 4. Microcomputer workstations--Health aspects. 5. Health. I. Sisson, Mark, 1953- II. Nicol, Jillian. III. Title.

RM725 .B692 2015
615.82  2015946726

*For my parents, who both worked very, very hard.*

## ALSO BY KATY BOWMAN

*Every Woman's Guide to Foot Pain Relief* (BenBella Books, 2011)

*Alignment Matters* (Propriometrics Press, 2013)

*Move Your DNA* (Propriometrics Press, 2014)

*Whole Body Barefoot* (Propriometrics Press, 2015)

# contents

AS REGULAR READERS of MarksDailyApple.com know, I'm one of the original fans of the standup desk movement that has really picked up steam in recent years. Several years ago at our Primal Blueprint headquarters in Malibu, CA, we rigged up some prehistoric primal standup desks by stacking together several varieties of USPS shipping boxes to raise monitors and keyboards. Today, each employee workstation has been outfitted with equipment specifically designed for "working out" on company time. Friends who drop in and see my setup (which includes a desk "kickstand" as described on page 42) have mentioned it looks like I'm typing emails while sitting on a pogo stick! Whatever, it's hard to deny the renewed flexibility and suppleness in my hip flexors.

Now many employees groove along, accumulating two to three miles of treadmill walking each day, in between periods of simply standing on a stationary treadmill belt or sitting down on a stool or regular chair. Meanwhile, mainstream media has embraced the hot tagline that "Sitting is the New Smoking." Progressive-minded large corporations are retrofitting cubicles with standup options, and millions of individuals working from home and even in dorm rooms are becoming more cognizant of the need to avoid prolonged stationary periods with their bodies hunched over keyboards.

I'm honored to write the foreword to Katy's book, as I believe she is the world leader in this burgeoning field of biomechanics and how it relates to optimal human development and health—not only when working, but also during physical activity, and even while relaxing or sleeping. Katy's presentations on biomechanics blend the "separate" fields of biological, physical, and kinesiology science with a practical, hands-on approach to working with real people. She also lives her message—writing, teaching, and maintaining a busy global travel schedule without sacrificing her body's need for movement.

When I initially reached out to Katy about collaborating on a solution to the "sitting is the new smoking" problem by promoting my beloved standup desks, I have to admit I was taken aback by her initial comments. "Is sitting the new smoking? Not really," countered Katy. "It's not as simple as trading a sitting desk for a standup desk. If you stand there all day in one position you'll be no better off than you were before…except you'll be more tired, stiff, and sore!"

Katy's view makes intuitive sense to me. Even with my enthusiastic adoption of standup working, I must admit I have a couple of "bailout" spots at my house where I grab my laptop and settle in with multiple pillows in my comfortable outdoor daybed structure (taking care to keep my spine in good alignment of course!), or perch on a simple stool at the kitchen counter for a change of pace. I felt guilty before talking to Katy, like I was cheating or simply didn't have the staying power yet of an all-day standup worker. Now I realize I'm just doing what my genes are calling for—variation in positioning and routine.

Indeed, we are challenged with a complex biomechanical problem here, for which there is no simple solution. I always reference the ancestral model when sorting through options to counter the health-compromising effects of high-tech life, and indeed we can reference the example of our ancestors in this case too. Most prehistoric hunter-gatherers likely lived a life that was wildly fluctuating in physical activity from day to day. They were generalists in every sense of the word, because their lives depended upon them possessing a variety of physical skills and abilities to navigate the ever-present challenges and dangers of primal life.

Today, in order to make an economic contribution to high-tech modern life, we've essentially been forced to become specialists. This is great for us when we need an electrician to remodel our bathroom or an orthopedic surgeon to scope our knee. However, we as individuals must recognize this discord, from an evolutionary perspective; from a physical, cellular perspective; and also from an intellectual perspective. Richard A. Heinlein, author of *Stranger in a Strange Land*, captured this sentiment memorably when he wrote, "A human being should be able to change a diaper, plan an invasion, butcher a hog, conn a ship, design a building, write a sonnet, balance accounts, build a wall, set a bone, comfort the dying, take orders, give orders, cooperate, act alone, solve equations, analyze a new problem, pitch manure, program a computer, cook a tasty meal, fight efficiently, die gallantly. Specialization is for insects."

As Katy will detail here, humans are designed for a fractal existence featuring an assortment of daily movement and physical challenges. And these genetically optimal physical challenges are not just the rote stuff like walking your two miles or cycling through your seven strength training stations at the gym, but spontaneous challenges that get your body moving in new and extraordinary ways.

And sorry to break it to you, folks, but being a fitness enthusiast, or even a serious competitive athlete, doesn't give you a free pass here. As breaking science has revealed with the so-called active couch potato syndrome, even those who follow a devoted schedule of daily workouts are not free from the disease risk of sedentary living when the majority of their days are spent commuting, working a desk job, and enjoying immobile leisure pursuits such as screen entertainment. Furthermore, even those with active jobs—for example, a lineman for the utility company, a building contractor, or a shipping and receiving agent— are generally engaged in repetitive tasks that only mobilize a fraction of their joints and muscles. And the grind of physical labor (particularly when using inefficient mechanics) can lead to assorted overuse injuries and health problems.

The solution here is not more visits to the gym or more miles on the road, or even installing a standup desk and carrying on. Every little step away from being sedentary helps, of course, but we need to mix things up a bit— make that a lot—in daily life. Be wary of routines, modern comforts, and all manner of sedentary momentum. If you enjoy your evening television programming, can you do a few sets of planks and squats while your eyes are glued to the digital stimulation? Will your office and company survive if you break free from your desk frequently to take phone calls or even personal meetings while cruising around the office courtyard?

Don't worry, there will be no shortage of ideas and even edicts presented here, but taking action is up to you. While at first it might seem like a hassle and an inconvenience to take the stairs instead of the elevators or to always park at the farthest spot in the lot instead of habitually trolling for the closest, pretty soon you will integrate new habits of this sort such that creative movement becomes second nature. Then, you will set a powerful example for your fellow humans who blithely scheme and strategize ways to elevate their lazy scorecards to world-class levels.

Let's leave specialization to the insects, and reject monotony, laziness, and dated social conventions. Instead, with some increased awareness and new tools and skills, you can start enjoying your hard-wired preference for an active, spontaneous, playful daily existence. Good luck with your journey!

Yours in health,
Mark Sisson, Malibu, CA

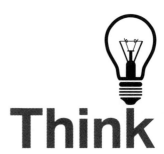

# Think

**chapter 1**

## SITTING ISN'T REALLY THE NEW SMOKING!

IF YOU HANG out on Internet health sites, chances are you've read a headline that screams something like "Sitting is the New Smoking!" These headlines imply that sitting, like smoking, is statistically associated with numerous health issues, including death from cardiovascular disease and cancer, and that it will take some time before we all wise up and quit.

As a long-time proponent of the Stop Sitting So Much campaign, I am thrilled that sitting is finally getting attention in the media. Research into diseases associated with sitting (like cancer) aren't new. The first article I ever read (in 1997) on sitting and cancer risk was published in 1993, which means scientists, at least somewhere, have known about this relationship for at least 20 years.

In light of sitting research and sit-less campaigns, healthy-minded individuals have been super motivated to get out of their chairs and onto physio balls, standing workstations, and tread-desks. The options to sit less are endless, so the notion that standing in one place is the solution to sitting so much reminds me of the joke about all accidents happening 15 miles from your home. "I read that all accidents happen within 15 miles of one's house, so I moved." Or, "I read that sitting kills, so now I'm afraid to stop standing."

As I explain more deeply in my book *Move Your DNA: Restore Your Health Through Natural Movement*, the sitting itself isn't really the problem; it is the repetitive use of a single position that makes us literally become ill in a litany of ways. For example, muscles will adapt to repetitive positioning by changing their cellular makeup, which in turn leads to less joint range of motion. This muscle and joint "stiffness" can lead to a stiffening of the arterial walls *within* these muscles. The positive news is that, because we've all been sitting (static) the same way for decades, changing our static positioning (i.e., standing more) can improve our health, as can moving intermittently throughout the day.

As a biomechanist, I help people understand that the shape of their body on the gross level (i.e., their posture) affects the shape of the cells themselves. In other words, the way you have been sitting has changed the tiny parts that make up your structure, like the shape and density of your bones, the length of your muscles and tendons, and the resting tension in your connective tissues. The adaptation to sitting on this deeper, cellular level means that reaping the benefits of "not sitting so much" requires more than just swapping one static position for another—it requires an entire overhaul of the way you think about and move your body.

> REAPING THE BENEFITS OF "NOT SITTING SO MUCH" REQUIRES MORE THAN JUST SWAPPING ONE STATIC POSITION FOR ANOTHER—IT REQUIRES AN ENTIRE OVERHAUL OF THE WAY YOU THINK ABOUT AND MOVE YOUR BODY.

Eventually the "all you need to do to fix yourself is to start standing" advice made me realize that a more thorough breakdown or explanation was needed—starting with the metaphor.

Sitting and smoking are different: sitting itself isn't the creator of ill effects the way smoking a cigarette is. Sitting—the position—is perfectly harmless when "consumed" appropriately. It's not like putting your butt into a chair makes you ill; as they say, "it's the dose that makes the poison." Language can also get us into trouble when we're seeking solutions, because we keep equating sitting with not moving, but in many cases, the physical effects of sitting are just as much created by repetitive geometry (always sitting in the same way) as they are by the metabolic changes that come with being sedentary. So sitting differently can improve your health in the same way that standing can—which is great news for the millions of people who aren't yet quite fit enough to stand for considerable amounts of time. Yes, even you—who want to change your risk profile for disease but feel trapped by your current physical limitations—can

**ANATOMY BIT**

Your arteries are arranged in a specific way to maximize pressure gradients and keep blood flow smooth, but this geometry changes with your posture. Prolonged alterations in arterial geometry can change the way blood flows through your tubes, creating scenarios where the loads to the vessel wall induce changes to the cells—causing them to go from *atheroprotective* (protective against the formation of plaque) to *atherogenic* (promoting the formation of plaque).

change how you sit and improve your health on a cellular level.

I'd be remiss if I didn't tease out how "standing" is not the simple, turnkey solution we might think it is. Every way of standing is not equal, and there are ways to stand that load your cells and create positive adaptations. What's the point of standing in a way that crushes your body in the same manner that sitting did?

The problem with equating sitting with smoking (or equating standing up with being the end-all solution) is that it oversimplifies the problem to be the act of sitting. Heralding standing still as the solution to sitting still perpetuates the problematic belief that there is a way we can consume a vast amount of stillness—whether it be sitting or standing—and still have the level of health necessary for a thriving quality of life.

My reason for writing this book is that, right now, you are probably super motivated to sit less, and I'd like to help you transition appropriately. In order to do that, you need a deeper prescription for sitting less than simply "standing more." Therefore, I've included the following four sections in this book:

- How to build a perfect workstation
- How to sit better
- How to stand better
- How to work out on company time!

The last section is a two-parter, because not only will I give you exercises to de-chair your body on your movement breaks, but I will also show how you can exercise your body while you are simultaneously working (you won't need extra time outside of work to do these exercises).

## RESEARCH CORNER

### SITTING AND CORONARY ARTERY CALCIFICATION

According to the Centers of Disease Control (CDC), coronary artery disease is the leading cause of death in the United States. The amount of sitting typically required for office work is associated with increased coronary artery calcification, an early marker for heart disease risk. One study, analyzing heart scans and accelerometer data (a device that measures how much you move) of more than 2,000 adults, found that each hour of sedentary time per day on average was associated with a 14 percent increase in coronary artery calcification burden. The association between calcification and sitting was independent of exercise activity and other traditional heart disease risk factors.

American College of Cardiology. (2015). Excess sitting linked to coronary artery calcification, an early indicator of heart problems. *ScienceDaily*, March 5, 2015. Retrieved online: sciencedaily.com/releases/2015/03/150305205959.htm.

## SCREEN TIME

I'd feel like a jerk if I didn't also mention that while sitting is indeed a risk factor for death and disease, so is screen time. Which means that even when you stand up, if you continue to look at a computer screen or smartphone all day, you haven't transitioned out of the danger zone as much as you'd like. Screen time and lack of movement are correlated, but they are separate variables and should be approached independently. Even if you've developed the habit of taking a daily walk, you still need to look at the frequency with which you're using your device (handheld or otherwise) and reduce it. Anyone who has been on a diet knows that starvation doesn't work. The most successful way to approach a change in diet is through small changes—cutting back on processed carbs or seeking organic produce instead of conventional, for example.

Here's your homework: Instead of resolving to throw your smart phone into the ocean, practice taking small breaks away from it. Pulling (tearing, ripping, etc.) yourself away from those addictive screens for a short time (three minutes) a dozen or so times a day is a habit you can cultivate. Needing your screen for work is one thing; being addicted to it is another. Use that tech break to take a three-minute walk or stretch. Bored? Don't check your email again. Just put the phone down and touch your toes instead. Standing in line at the bank? Stand on one leg and practice some of the steps to alignment discussed in Chapter 5. Go to the bathroom "alone" (read: without your tech-buddy) for a change and focus on how you get down onto and up off the toilet. There is health to be found in three-minute sessions. You can find it.

chapter 2

## THE SINGLE BEST ERGONOMIC POSITION? NO SUCH THING!

MODERN ERGONOMICS IS not the scientific pursuit of what is best for the human body, but the scientific pursuit of how the human body can be positioned (in *one* position, for eight or more hours at a time) for the purpose of returning to work the next day, and then the next and the next and the next. Before you apply ergonomic data to your workstation, consider this: *Finding an "optimal working position" is not about your long-term health as much as it is about your production value over a short period of employable time.* This isn't to say that your office's ergonomics expert doesn't have your best interests at heart, but that there's a broader perspective to be

**ANATOMY BIT**

According to the *Journal of Occupational and Environmental Medicine*, health care expenditures are nearly 50 percent greater for workers who report high levels of stress.

considered. There really isn't a healthy way for the body to sit for long periods of time; there is only a way to sit that loads the parts damaged by chronic sitting in a less damaging way.

Therapeutically, we tend to solve pain problems by seeking a "better" body position than our current one. But the problem with our bodies is rarely the position we hold them in; the problem is the high frequency at which we are in a repetitive position. Being in a single position repetitively, as we have been when chair-sitting (or computer-using, or car-driving, or stressing), means that there are an infinite number of other positions going unused.

For decades, researchers have been trying to figure out the best way to organize the body for optimal performance at the office. The underlying flaw in much of the research—or at least in the presentation of the research—is that it fails to highlight the *use of a single position* as the problem. Our quest to find an optimal position for stillness will always be frustrated by the problems inherent in a lack of movement. Fortunately, in light of new understanding regarding the importance of all-day movement as opposed to exercise buried in a mostly sedentary day, there is a new trend in health research across the board: to look at the physiological and biomechanical effects of the sitting behavior.

I've brought all of this up because I want you to understand why I've chosen to write a book on why the *sedentary desk*—whether it be a sitting or standing one—is the problem. If we keep trying to solve the "what's the best way to be in front of my computer" problem, we'll miss that the answer is "as little as possible." That all being said, you still need to work, be in front of your computer, and commute with regularity. But our lack of knowing (yet) how to solve the problem shouldn't keep us from discussing the actual problem. The fact that we must work can be considered as we try to figure out how to use more of our bodies' ranges of motion, to prevent our muscles and other body tissues from atrophying in this movement drought.

There are evidence-based ways to sit and stand better, but the conditions that make these positions better for you are limited in scope. Which is why in addition to making postural adjustments, which introduce new body loads and require different muscles to work, you also need to move more throughout the day—*throughout* being the key term. The newest research shows that you can be active (as in, faithfully completing your daily workout at the gym or logging "10 miles ran today" on your marathon-training program) and still be sedentary (as in, commuting back and forth each day to your desk job and consuming extensive digital entertainment in your leisure hours).

OUR QUEST TO FIND AN OPTIMAL POSITION FOR STILLNESS WILL ALWAYS BE FRUSTRATED BY THE PROBLEMS INHERENT IN A LACK OF MOVEMENT.

Let's work to solve the problem by not just getting up and out of our chairs, but by creating intermittent movement—both on the large and small scale—while still getting our business/work done. As you proceed through the next sections about workstations, sitting, standing, and doing clever exercises in the office, always keep the big-picture goal in mind that these optimal setups are really way stations to flow through over the course of the workday.

## IS YOUR JOB STRESSING YOU OUT?

When you're stressed, an alarm goes off in your brain to which your body responds, preparing your body for defensive action. If you work at a circus as a tiger trainer, this lifesaving fight-or-flight mechanism probably comes in handy. But if you're busy dumping muscle-tensing, tunnel-vision-making, respiration-and-heart-rate-increasing hormones into your bloodstream every time you open your email or every time the office jerk strolls by your door, job stress can easily be breaking down your body tissues, escalating your risk of injury and disease. The solution: Instead of (only) adding a new workstation and exercises to your routine, see where work stress can be eliminated.

Does checking your email fill you with a sense of dread? Don't check your email 20 times a day (read: 20 biochemical dumps and 20 clenches of the jaw and neck muscles). Add an automatic response to emails: "To increase my productivity, I check and respond to emails twice a day at these times _____." Pick the times that work best for you according to your schedule. Add a line like, "For urgent matters, please call me directly at _____." Unless it's the phone that drives you mad. Then, add a message to your voicemail saying that you only check your phone messages once a day and for faster service, send an email! Whatever your preference, you can ask people to accommodate you. Your health and productivity depend on it!

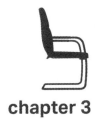

chapter 3

## BUILDING THE PERFECT WORKSTATION FOR YOU

IF SOMEONE ASKED your position at work, you would give them the title of your job—but couldn't "sitting" also be a valid answer? Of course it could, which is why you're reading this book on standing workstations. In fact, this isn't (only) a section on sitting vs. standing workstations; it's about all the body positions in between and around chair-sitting and standing that you can assume while working.

Most people are familiar with the term "form" as it applies to exercise and working out, but our use of form is very linear. If we were magically set free from the cages of our modern, agricultural, post–Industrial Revolution, tech-based culture and transported back to earlier times where we had to find food and water daily, build shelters, and carry our worldly possessions with our arms, our bodies would be exposed to a constant stream of work and variety. We'd be walking on varying terrain, with all sorts of random angles and grades under our feet; we'd be sitting at different heights, in different ways, on a wide range of objects; we'd be using our arms and backs in whatever ways were necessary. So clearly, to think of standing as the only alternative to sitting in a chair is very limiting when it comes to optimizing our body's function in daily life.

The key to finding health through the use of alternative workstations is to make sure your setups are as fluid as possible. The more time you spend at a "fixed" station—even a super fancy setup with a five-star rating—the closer you will be to exactly where you were when you were sitting all day. Sure, standing is great after a decade spent sitting, but without the refreshment of your mechanosensors (tiny sensors in your cells), your body will just begin a new set of adaptations to your new static position. And it's important to note that *adaptations* do not necessarily equal *improvements*.

Let's say you spent every last dollar and free minute you had getting this book. There's no money left to buy your dream desk setup or time to shop for it. Here's a secret: If you sit cross-legged in your chair, right now as you're reading this, you'll be doing your body better because you're loading different parts. Don't want to (or can't) cross both legs at the same time? Try one ankle over your opposite knee. After a few minutes, switch to the other. Do you work frequently from a laptop? Sit on a pillow on the floor with your legs out in a V-position and set your computer on a stack of books. Sit cross-legged with your computer on the floor or on a box, lie on your stomach, stand at a counter, or at a desk— all within the space of an hour, if it suits you. Get what I'm saying? The combinations and permutations of a workstation are *endless*. Sometimes we get so fixated on "doing it the right way" that we forget "the right way" is "as many different ways as you can."

## MECHANOSENSING

Cells in your body have parts within them that have the specific function of sensing your mechanical environment (i.e., how your cells are squished in response to the forces created through moving and position). In a process called *mechanotransduction*, the distortion in the shape of these cells is turned into chemical signals that create adaptations on the cellular and tissue levels. Imagine mechanosensors as fluid-filled balloons, then imagine squeezing the sides together— the ends would bulge out. Or if you pulled the ends away from each other, the middle section would compress the fluid inward. The distortion of the mechanosensor (the cell's structural change and the resulting movement of the fluid inside of it) is mechanical input—information that a cell can use to adapt. The way we adapt depends on how we—our cells, really—are deformed. But it's not only the deformation of the cell that signals a particular behavior; the *frequency* of cell-stimulation is just as if not more important than the load (cell-deforming squeeze or pull) itself. If you want to make your body stronger, you have to move. Period.

While assorted creative and comfortable positions sound

## RESEARCH CORNER

### MECHANOTRANSDUCTION IN ACTION:
### OFFICE A$$ IS A REAL THING

It's not only your pants that stretch when you sit; the cells that make up your butt-flesh deform as the weight of your pelvis presses into the mass that you sit upon. Can you imagine how a ball of clay would spread out if you were to sit on it? A similar spreading of the cells that make up your butt tissue occurs in three directions, and creates a particular signal within these cells via a process called mechanotransduction. Remember when I said that an adaptation isn't always an improvement? Here's a little mechanotransduction in action: Research has shown that sustained deformation of a fat cell can lead the cell to produce lipids (more fat) at a faster rate. What's this mean for you? It means GET UP.

Al-Dirini, R.M.A., Reed, M.P., & Thewlis, D. (2015). Deformation of the gluteal soft tissues during sitting. *Clinical Biomechanics,* May 22. Retrieved online: clinbiomech.com/article/S0268-0033(15)00144-8/abstract

Shoham, N., Gottlieb, R., Shaharabani-Yosef, O., Zaretsky, U., Benayahu, D., & Gefen, A. (2011). Static Mechanical Stretching Accelerates Lipid Production in 3T3-L1 Adipocytes by Activating the MEK Signaling Pathway. *American Journal of Physiology - Cell Physiology,* October.

enticing, you may face certain constraints in a traditional office environment. Don't worry—we accept that the real challenge is making your body healthier while respecting workplace norms and providing solutions that fall in line with acceptable office behavior. If you follow the guidelines in this book, especially the alignment markers, you'll find that you can expose your body to many different cellular loads while you work in the standard, "upright" way.

Since you'll be wanting to adjust all your workstations, I'm happy to point out that the standing workstation is a pretty basic concept—move your keyboard and screen to a higher platform that doesn't require you to sit in a chair. You can create one quickly and inexpensively with stuff you probably already have. Setting your computer up on a counter or bar in your home, flipping a box upside down on your regular desk, and grabbing a simple plastic stool from a home supply store creates a standing workstation in an instant. I've also found perusing thrift stores for cool bookshelves and adaptable furniture to be quite fruitful. Architect's tables and other specialized products that allow you to adjust the height (including low platforms that enable you to sit on the floor and still have a wide and flat workspace) are also options.

I've been writing and lecturing on dynamic stations for about five years now, and many people who have converted to a dynamic setup have been kind enough to submit pictures to help spark your creative juices and show you how easy this transition can be (see next page).

Ranging from quickly fashioned to self-manufactured to pre-fashioned for exactly the purpose of standing at work, you can see the sky is the limit when it comes to creativity.

## STANDING WORKSTATION KITS

Pre-fab stand-up kits are reliably stable and safe for office use, which can make transitioning at work simpler if you need approval from your supervisor or human resources department. (I don't imagine that your HR department would be super thrilled by your 40-pound monitor wobbling on top of the upside-down laundry basket you brought from home.) The only drawback, if you can call it that, is that a fixed setup might limit your options when your body is calling to

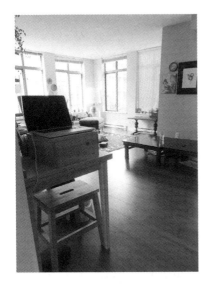

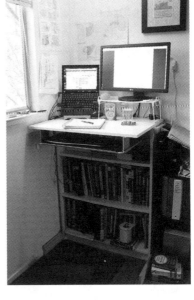

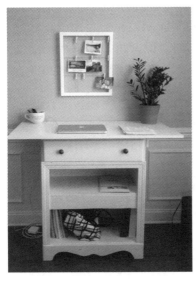

sit down. Yes, there are times when sitting is fine. In fact, if you stand the bulk of the day, sitting breaks are helpful. If your transition to a standing station makes your old office chair obsolete, consider a low-profile stool or a kickstand (read more on these in Chapter 4) that slides under your desk when not in use.

## IS THERE A PERFECT KEYBOARD?

If you've ever been in a cast for a couple of months, then you know that when you take it off, your tissues have adapted to being in a fixed position. A casted limb is an extreme example of static positioning, but this phenomenon—your tissues adapting to match your most frequented position—is occurring on a smaller scale all of the time. While your arms are not exactly in a cast, your neck, shoulders, elbows, and wrists are repetitively exposed to the same joint configurations, which promotes significant atrophy in both the muscles and the tissues that connect them.

The keyboard of your computer is often blamed for forcing your hands into a bad position, but maintaining or frequenting any single position over a period of time will result in the same thing: a repetitive-use injury. Rather than trying to find the keyboard that offers a single, static, "optimal hand position," find a keyboard that offers you an

WHEN "COMPUTERING," YOUR NECK, SHOULDERS, ELBOWS, AND WRISTS ARE REPETITIVELY EXPOSED TO THE SAME JOINT CONFIGURATIONS, WHICH PROMOTES SIGNIFICANT ATROPHY IN BOTH THE MUSCLES AND THE TISSUES THAT CONNECT THEM.

**ANATOMY BIT**

**The upper body wins! (or does it?)** According to the Occupational Health and Safety Administration, 33 percent of all work-related injuries are musculoskeletal disorders. Of these disorders, most occur in the upper part of the body (hands, elbows, shoulder, and neck).

assortment of positions, and use them!

The newest keyboards on the market can splay (one half slides away from the other) at varying degrees. Some fully separate into two pieces. You can also find keyboards that can be adjusted to use different degrees of wrist extension. (What is wrist extension? Reach your arms out in front of you, palms down, in zombie fashion. Now, move your hands back toward you, hinging at the wrist. The motion that makes the angle between the hand and lower arm smaller is called wrist extension.) You'll be surprised to find that any change to your board will require a learning curve that can be frustrating at times. The good news about all those misspelled words is that learning new motor programs means you're working different muscles (or the same muscles, differently). Changing your muscle-use pattern on simple tasks like typing does the same thing for prevention of repetitive-use injuries that cross-training does for your overall athletic performance.

Most upper body parts are desperately under-loaded and under-utilized in comparison to the  legs (for info on how our upper bodies are similar to the flopped-over fins of captive orcas, read *Move Your DNA*). The shoulder's range of motion is not only mind-blowing, it is mind-blowingly underused. The bonus of a keyboard that separates is that, if you wanted, you could work with your hands at a greater distance from each other than the typical placement found in offices the world over. In order to widen your hands, the bones making up your shoulder joint have to change position, which is a good thing for the muscles, blood vessels, and nerves in this area. Issues like shoulder impingement syndrome (bursitis, bicep tendon tear, etc.) and thoracic outlet syndrome are brought about by insane amounts of stillness surrounding even more insane frequencies of tiny movement (like clicking your computer mouse).

## RESEARCH CORNER

While it might be tough to walk and chew gum at the same time, what about other things, like recalling emails? In one study, 18 subjects were given a text and emails to read while they either sat (control group) or walked on a treadmill desk. Ten minutes later, everyone was given a quiz regarding what they had read; those who were walking answered correctly a higher percentage of time.

Labonté-LeMoyne, É., Santhanam, R., Léger, P., Courtemanche, F., Fredette, M., & Sénécal, S. (2015). The Delayed Effect of Tread-mill Desk Usage On Recall and Attention. *Computers in Human Behavior, 46,* 1-5.

## TREADMILL DESKS

Movement is king, and if there is a workstation that allows you to move and work, then that has to be queen, right? I believe there are indisputable benefits to treadmill desks; they allow you to keep moving in a way that's great for your mind, metabolism, and circulatory system (read more about veins on pages 84–86). However, as a studier of natural movement, I also believe that there are many yet-to-be measured variables—potential drawbacks—that may appear slight but that, over time, could create profound effects on our physiology and health.

## TREADMILLS AND GAIT

To move through this world, you can either push backward using muscular force to move forward (think of a paddle pushing back against the water to move a canoe forward through the water), or lean and fall forward, using gravity to do the work, your weight pulling you toward the ground in front of you. Our natural, reflex-driven gait involves a big posterior push-off. This is a complex muscular event that uses the lateral hip muscles, glutes, and hamstrings. Walking or running in this manner maintains your torso's uprightness, keeps your spine stable, loads the pelvic and hip bones optimally (strengthening them where they should be strengthened), and keeps frequent loads to your knees and hips to a magnitude they can handle well.

You can probably guess what's coming next, yes?

This posterior push-off (rowing action) of the leg requires the ground to be fixed. The belt on a treadmill is not fixed. In fact, it's already moving in the direction you'd want your leg to be going, which means you need an entirely different way of walking to deal with a treadmill. When you are on a treadmill, your body, instead of firing muscles to push back, is forced to catch up to the moving belt—meaning you have to actively lift your legs up in front of you. While the walk may look the same, the pattern of muscular activation involved in walking on a treadmill is entirely different from that involved in walking over land.

The gait we are forced to use while walking on a treadmill is a recipe for future injury, the ingredient list being one part repetitive hip flexion (a movement pattern people visit a physical therapist to learn how to undo in the event of particular injuries and diseases) and one part the repetitive and excessive blow to the legstuffs (foot, knee, and hip tissues) used to catch and cushion millions of tiny falls.

By using a treadmill, not only are you missing out on the many benefits of a natural gait (like strong glutes, which help support your pelvic floor), but you're actually creating tiny negative outcomes that over the long-term could add up to overworked knees, hips, and lower back tissues, just to name a few. (This goes for non-office treadmill use as well. I really hate to be the one to say it, but treadmills are to walking as McDonald's is to whole food. They look similar to the untrained eye but the differences to our physiology are measurable. And, P.S., if you're wondering how your family and friends feel every time you point out that the food they eat is not compatible with their human machinery, it's the same way you are feeling RIGHT NOW. It's difficult to wrap your brain around something so commonly accepted and seemingly benign being not great, right? Wrap your message in compassion; this stuff is pretty mind-blowing. The end.)

Considering both the mechanical side effects and the metabolic ones begs the question: "Is it still better to be walking on a treadmill than not at all?" And I don't know if there's a

way to derive the answer. It just depends on what outcome
you are after and the health issues you may already be experiencing. The final outcome of a pros and cons list depends on
who's doing the pro-ing and con-ing.

If you're experiencing metabolic issues, then yes, all-day
movement is going to be in your favor. But if you're currently
experiencing musculoskeletal issues of the hips, low back,
pelvic floor, or knee joint,
then logging millions of
hip-flexing steps could
exacerbate your issues. The
solution we are after is to
not just fix the current issue
(too little body use) but to
fix it in a way that doesn't
hinder necessary move-
ments needed for health in
the future. This is a tricky negotiation and it's also why these
details matter.

> TREADMILL WALKING HAS PROS
> AND CONS. BEST ADVICE IS
> DON'T LOG THESE MILES TOWARD
> YOUR DAILY WALKING. YOU STILL
> HAVE TO GET OUT AND MOVE
> OVER GROUND FOR OPTIMAL
> BIOLOGICAL FUNCTION.

If you've decided on a treadmill desk, the best advice I can
offer is this: Don't log these miles toward your daily walking.
Sure, you might have walked eight miles every day (and
bravo, by the way), but this way of walking might not leave
you with the muscle distribution the human body requires
for optimal biological function. Meaning, you still need to
log your necessary miles—over ground—once you're done
walking on your treadmill.

Also, you'll want to build small actual walks across the earth
into your workday—walk for three minutes every half hour
of your eight-hour workday, and you'll have been moving for

an extra forty-eight minutes every day. (I cannot even tell you how much these three-minute "health" breaks add up. They really do!) Spend your lunch hour and breaks in motion (see the next chapter for moves that restore parts rather than break them down), and you'll be doing even better.

## SOFTWARE AND LIGHT

Your eyes are constantly adjusting to your environment by shortening or lengthening muscles. These muscles change the shape of your eyes' lenses in order to focus on the scenery you take in. But the effects of the environment don't just stop with muscular lengthening and contraction within the eyes; your eyes are also a gateway to your brain. In addition to seeing for seeing's sake, your eyes gather sensory data regarding time of day, for example. As the light winds down, this change in wavelength kick-starts a hormonal cycle that prepares the body for rest. Humans don't need to expend energy maintaining a separate organ whose sole purpose is to "tell time." Your eyes have evolved to handle this function as well. But what happens when you remove the biological catalyst (slowly fading light) from the biological system? What happens then?

While the masses might turn their "work computers" off at 5:00, often "fun computer" time starts at 5:01. In fact, there's a pretty good chance that most of you are still looking at one, two, or several different device screens right up until bedtime. And then wondering why it's difficult to go to sleep.

Melatonin, a hormone secreted by the pituitary gland, is responsible for regulating sleep and the reproductive cycle. Any light that you are exposed to after sunset can suppress

## RESEARCH CORNER

If you've ever taken a long flight, you're probably aware that long bouts of sitting affect blood flow in the legs. Research has shown that the flow of the main artery of the legs (femoral artery) was impaired as much as 50 percent in just one hour. Over a three-hour period, subjects taking a gentle five-minute walk at 30, 90, and 150 minutes were able to keep the blood flowing well through the lower legs.

Thosar, S.S., Bielko, S.L., Mather, K.J., Johnston, J.D., & Wallace, J.P. (2015). Effect of Prolonged Sitting and Breaks in Sitting Time on Endothelial Function. *Medicine and Science in Sports and Exercise, 47(4)*, 843-849.

melatonin (which is important to consider as we dwell in a night-lighting culture), but blue light (the kind emitted by digital screens and most light bulbs) is especially stimulating.

Alongside growing consideration for how light affects our biology has come the development of in-office light bulbs and software modifications that can change the variables of light we expose ourselves to and therefore adaptations we experience (see Appendix for a list of light-altering products). And let us not forget that we can always choose to eliminate and/or reduce the duration we're exposed to artificial light altogether, by establishing natural light in our office (i.e., moving the

SINCE THE LIGHT BULB WAS INVENTED SO RECENTLY IN THE EVOLUTIONARY TIMELINE, HUMANS ARE ABSOLUTELY UNACCUSTOMED TO DIGITAL-LIGHT STIMULATION AFTER DARK. MIND YOUR OWN ECOSYSTEM AND MELLOW THINGS OUT AFTER DARK.

desk near a window) and by turning off our devices, or at least making a concerted effort to restrict their use (and the brightness of the screen) after the sun sets each day. You'll find that turning off your device even for a couple of hours

## NIGHT-LIGHTING

"Natural transitions between light and darkness influence the biology and behavior of many organisms. What happens when humans introduce light into darkness?" – Michael Salmon.

Once, on the Yucatan peninsula, I participated in a biologist group assisting the release of day-old sea-turtle hatchlings into the ocean. Turtles typically emerge from their shells at night and walk toward the ocean—recognizable by its glimmer or reflection of the moon—hop in the water and get going on their way. As you can imagine, human intervention is not necessary for this process to run smoothly. So, what were we doing there?

If you've ever vacationed on the Cancun strip you've probably noticed the barrage of hotels running the length of the beaches, and it's along these same beaches that turtles have been building nests for eons. Unfortunately, with hotels come continuous illumination, especially problematic for new turtle hatchlings genetically programed to "seafind" by responding reflexively to the light cast by the water. In night-lighted areas, baby turtles were found to walk in circles, confused by the increased sources of light—some dying due to prolonged exposure and some dying after ending up in the hotel's chlorinated swimming pools.

We forget that humans, like turtles, are animals that have particular requirements for optimal biological function. Sleeping patterns,

**NIGHT-LIGHTING (CON'T)**

fertility patterns, and many other biological behaviors are known to be affected by the presence of artificial light after the sun has gone down.

Light bulbs have been with us since the 1800s and used heavily for fewer than 100 years, making "night-lighting" less than a seconds-old habit to our physiology, comparatively speaking. We, like all animals, are absolutely unaccustomed to digital-light stimulation after dark. If you're experiencing issues related to melatonin, I strongly suggest you evaluate your relationship with the light input experienced by your own personal ecosystem.

a day has multiple benefits, such as eliminating the invisible (light) as well as the tangible ("device postures") and allowing more time for movement. Again, solutions to office-related health issues have less to do with the office/work itself and more to do with our all-day relationship with technology.

## MONKEY BAR

I, for one, love monkey business. I'm lucky enough to have built-in monkey bars in my home office, but adding this feature to your office is as simple as getting a portable chin-up bar to plop in your doorway when needed. In the same way your legs should stay strong enough to carry the weight of the body, so should your arms. Which isn't to say that you need to be doing a bunch of pull-ups for fitness's sake, but that even supported (meaning your feet are still on the ground) hanging gives you an instantaneous whole-body makeover that can generously provide a heap of loads—the

## RESEARCH CORNER

The public should, indeed, know more about health issues where light is a factor. Unfortunately, in the scope of the number of important environmental factors that need research, night-lighting is far along on the list and research is moving much more slowly than it should. For a great overview of "where science is" on the matter, I suggest reading a review article by Ron Chepesiuk—"**Missing the Dark: Health Effects of Light Pollution.**"

Chepesiuk, R. (2009). Missing The Dark: Health Effects of Light Pollution. *Environmental Health Perspectives, 117(1)*, A20-A27.

necessary physical deformation of your body's cells—that you're missing out on while remaining sedentary in your office.

Certainly a hang-on bar is not standard office fare, but that doesn't mean that it shouldn't be. Yes, it might appear like you're goofing off at first, but I'll bet that if you're the keeper of the company chin-up bar, your office will be the popular hangout for those needing an oxygen infusion break!

## WHAT IF YOU ALREADY STAND ALL DAY?

If you're a massage therapist or cook, or in any of the hundreds of other

### ANATOMY BIT

Light exposure can be broken into three categories: duration (the period of time over which you're exposed to light), quantity (the intensity or concentration of light you are exposed to), and quality (the wavelength or "color" reaching the surface of the eye). Blue and yellow light are examples of a quality of light.

professions that require you to be on your feet all day, this book is still for you. Remember, sitting isn't really the issue; it's always sitting. Standing all day long, or moving in the same patterns, can give you aches and pains (a sign of body breakdown) similar to those found in your typical cubicle-dweller. Instead of focusing on the workstation, focus on using alignment points, doing corrective exercises, and switching to minimal footwear (as explained on pages 56–59). You can also use the floor more (instead of a chair). Sitting on the ground instead of in a chair will bring unique joint and muscle use to your ankles, knees, hips, and torso, and contribute to improved overall well-being. Even if you stand a lot when you work, you may be sitting in a chair more than you realize when you examine your behavior throughout the day.

> HANGING GIVES YOU AN INSTANTANEOUS WHOLE-BODY MAKEOVER THAT CAN GENEROUSLY PROVIDE A HEAP OF LOADS YOU'RE MISSING OUT ON WHILE BEING SEDENTARY IN YOUR OFFICE.

## ADJUSTABLE WORKSTATIONS

The best workstation is one that gives you endless options (okay, how about at least two?). If there is one thing health experts agree on, it's that we need to move more. Even if your version of "move more" is created by changing your static positioning a few times throughout the day and moving a lot during short breaks in between positions, you're a heck of a lot better off than you would be in one fixed position all day long.

In the end, it is most helpful to think of every workstation (even if it's the standard, no frills, seated one you've had for the last decade) as an adjustable one; simply changing the way you sit can change your health for the better. Of course I want you to sit less, but I also want you to feel good about taking small steps. We can get so overwhelmed by all the ways we could improve that we feel paralyzed—we feel that if we don't do everything perfectly all at once, we're taking a step backward. This is why I am telling you right now that simply adjusting one body part (as you're about to learn) can change things drastically.

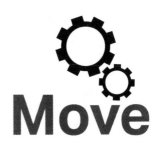

# Move

**chapter 4**

## SITTING WELL

SO, LET'S SAY that you haven't finished reading this book and you have no money to spend on even the most inexpensive version of a standing workstation (a crate flipped over on a table). Can you still change something, right now, to improve your health? The answer is yes.

If you weren't around in the 1920s, you might have missed the progression of furniture. Once straight-backed and stiff-seated, couches have gone uber-soft and car seats have gone bucket. I suppose we've evolved our furniture construction in the name of comfort, luxury, and technological "progress." But because our body shape adapts to the shape of the furniture we frequent, we, going forward, search out furniture shapes that disturb our current physiology the least. Thus we create a destructive cycle in which our culture influences our bodies, which in turn influence our culture.

Our grandparents walked and labored more than we do, and likewise we have moved more than the younger generation, which has had touch screens and computers since birth. Just like a 70-year-old woman who has worn high heels her entire life can no longer go barefoot lest she tear her shortened Achilles tendons, neither can most of us sit in a straight-backed chair for very long without soon experiencing discomfort. Our slouches feel natural to our unnaturally shaped bodies.

Sitting on a tucked-under pelvis places constant pressure on the sacrum (the triangular bone at the base of the spine) that can negatively impact the health of the pelvis, pelvic floor (the muscles that fill in the bottom of your pelvis and are, essentially, the basement of your entire torso), and spine. Adjusting your pelvis instantly changes the mechanical environment of your sacroiliac (SI) joint, your pelvis, and your lumbar spine. In the short term this adjustment can lead to a decrease in back or tailbone pain, and in the long term, it can improve the functions of the pelvis—including the fun ones.

In order to make adjustments without creating inappropriate muscle tension patterns, you must have a zero-rise chair; that is, one with a horizontal rather than angled sitting surface. Seats that are lower in the back force you to actively arch your back to accomplish this pelvic adjustment. Let's begin our adjustments by finding a flat-seated chair (a kitchen chair is usually flat) or fill in your bucket seat with a

**COMMUTERS**

Whether you drive your car to get to the office or your car is your office, you can make the ride better on your body by filling in your bucket seat and adjusting how you sit.

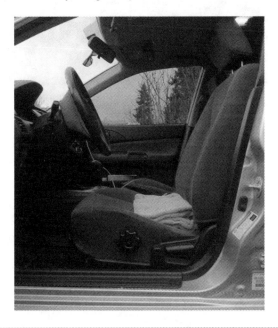

rolled towel to create a horizontally level surface (see picture above).

Start by sitting close to the edge of a chair; this will help you roll your pelvis forward. By forward I mean that the top ridge of your pelvis—commonly referred to as your hip bones—should move toward your knees, a shift that (conveniently) lifts the tailbone away from the chair.

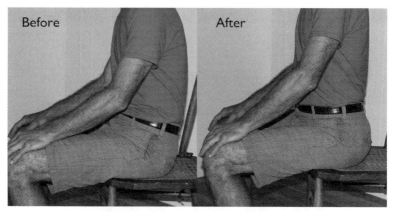

Before and after pelvic alignment

If your body is tight, you may have limited mobility at the hip joints, so for greater forward motion, sit on a folded and rolled bath towel.

A towel or any other "bolstering" apparatus will create a curve that will assist you in the forward tipping of your

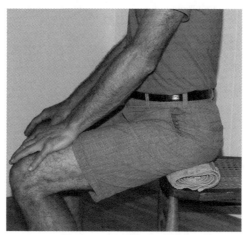

Sitting on rolled towel

pelvis. It's also a great way to highlight the undesirable sensation of tucking (the backward motion of the top of the pelvis)—you'll have an exaggerated "tucking" alarm all day!

## BALL-CHAIRS

Many people have transitioned from a chair to a physio/ stability ball. This transition comes with many benefits, as the decreased stability can promote greater core work and fidgeting—one way to keep on moving throughout the day. However, sitting on a ball is still sitting, and there's nothing about sitting on a ball that forces you to use your core; you can still slouch quite comfortably! To make over your ball-sitting, incorporate the same untucking motion (yes, a bit easier on the ball!) throughout the day, and make sure that your hips are not closer to the floor than your knees are.

### RESEARCH CORNER

Health is not only about calories, but if you're looking for a way to measure if you're working more, looking at calories expended is a simple way. Whether it's the lack of a back rest on the ball (to do the work naturally done by your stabilizing muscles), or the fact that it can move, one study found that subjects sitting on an exercise ball expended a little over four calories more per hour as compared to subjects sitting in a chair. I know four calories an hour doesn't seem like a lot, but if you think in terms of years, those four calories an hour are the equivalent to 2.5 pounds a year.

Beers, E.A., Roemmich, J.N., Epstein, L.H., et al. (2008). Increasing Passive Energy Expenditure During Clerical Work. *European Journal of Applied Physiology, 103(3)*, 353-360.

## IN SEARCH OF THE PERFECT CHAIR

I'm often asked for my recommendation for the best office chair, to which I have no good reply. What makes a chair good is the frequency with which you choose not to use it. Most of the problems with sitting are related to the perpetual stillness, not the position itself. That being said, many times people are looking for a chair that makes their_____ (fill in the blank) feel better. I suggest that you put your search efforts and spending dollars towards improving your musculoskeletal health through corrective exercise and alignment, and not towards a device that makes your tissue weaknesses less uncomfortable. Discomfort is nature's way of letting you know that something is wrong. And again, it's not necessarily the way you've been sitting that's hurting you (although yes, the way you sit can certainly give rise to problems) but the heaps and heaps of time you have spent sitting.

> WHAT MAKES A CHAIR GOOD IS THE FREQUENCY WITH WHICH YOU CHOOSE NOT TO USE IT. SPEND YOUR ENERGY ON IMPROVING YOUR MUSCULOSKELETAL HEALTH, NOT ON A DEVICE THAT MAKES YOUR TISSUE WEAKNESSES LESS UNCOMFORTABLE.

## DITCH THE CHAIR AND CONSIDER A SEAT

What is a chair, exactly? If both my kitchen (straight-back, hard-seated, four-legged) chair and my La-Z-Boy (essentially a full-body pillow on a frame) chair belong in the same category, then the word chair may not be the most useful one. Perhaps a better word, especially in light of the many options

**SQUATTING WORKSTATION?**

I once got a question on Facebook that asked, "Is a squatting work-station awesome or ridiculous?" Maybe a little of both! If you can sustain a squat without struggle or tensions that put your feet to sleep, then great. But squatting for a long period of time (like the dura-tion of a workday) is just as unnatural as sitting or standing. Taking a few squat breaks per day—now *that's* a good idea. Full disclo-sure: I have a squatty potty and a Twitter app on my iPhone and I'm not afraid to use both—at the same time. Frankly—and I think we've established that I'm comfortable being frank—one way that I've reduced my work time (I have small children) is to get done tiny tasks like returning emails and delegating items to my staff while on my "squatting workstation." I'm already just sitting there, and by blending these activities—*in a squat!*—I can shave off time spent sitting or standing in front of my computer, which gives me more time to be outdoors. (Note: I only recommend using your device on the commode if it can afford you some non-screen time at a different time. If you're taking a screen break from your work computer to play video games, then you're not really doing your body good. If this is you, see the sidebar on page 8 for my recommendation to go screen-free in the bathroom.)

now available, is seat. Anything you can rest your bottom on is a seat, and just as you can walk or stand in an endless series of joint configurations, so can you take a seat.

As you transition away from the traditional office chair, you'll find that you still want and need to rest on something. Is a chair your only option? Nope. Consider an alternative-to-a-chair seat that provides you with a different geometrical experience while still letting you sit. High (or low, for that matter) stools and body "kickstands"—essentially a single-legged device with a seat that allows you to rest while it kinda sorta supports you—are excellent, low-profile options to keep at any desk for use as necessary.

# chapter 5

# STANDING WELL

WHETHER AT A standing desk or in one of the hundreds of lines you will stand in this year, you can practice standing in a way that uses more muscles actively. Your body is a coping machine. It adapts well by quickly changing its cellular structure to reduce the energy output necessary to accomplish a task. For many people, standing is a passive activity; they arrange their skeletons with thrusts and bends to allow the resting tensions in connective tissues to bear the weight of the body. Awesome—who wants to be spending all that energy standing around? Only, here's the thing with adaptations: They are not necessarily for the long-term betterment of the body but the short term. Which means that the changes that allow you to stand *sans* muscle force can damage that connective tissue, and the parts that would otherwise be supporting the body will gradually lose function. Which means that thrusting your pelvis forward when you stand, which allows tension in the quads and psoas (a long muscle running between the spine just below the rib cage and the top of the thigh—on both sides of your body—attaching to all your lumbar vertebrae and spinal discs along the way) to hold you up, also takes the job of holding you up away from the butt and core muscles.

Also, if you stand in one place for very long—six to eight hours a day—these passive positions can do long-term damage to structures that don't adapt well. Bone and muscle you can train to restore. Ligaments? Not so much. All that rib thrusting (more below) can overstretch ligaments between vertebrae, and all that quad tension can weaken the structures in your knees.

The following is an eight-part checklist to help you stand better—meaning this arrangement uses greater muscular force to keep you in place, and decreases loads to the foot arches, knee ligaments, and lower back associated with long-term body damage.

By going through these steps you'll be checking and re-arranging the alignment markers that make for better whole-body use while standing at your workstations:

## STEP 1: FEET FORWARD
Align the outside edges of the feet with a straight edge, like a book or the edge of a yoga mat. (You're not actually lining

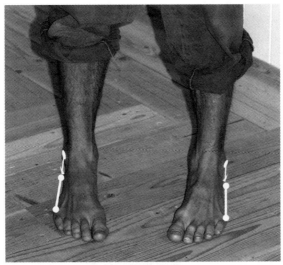

Feet forward

up the edge of each foot, but the two points shown in the pic: one is located by dropping an imaginary vertical line to the floor from the lateral edge of your ankle bone, and two is at the most lateral piece of foot bone before your pinky toe starts. It's okay if the edges of your feet look curved when they're lined up. Most people's are.)

Why? When standing still, this position optimizes the leverage of the foot-arch-making muscles in the feet and hips. Later, in step 6, you'll learn to rotate your thighs, and you won't be able to do it unless your feet are "neutral." Because you'll be on your feet for a long time, you'll want the muscles supporting your structure "on" and active.

Your lower leg turns out for many reasons: excessive sitting and footwear use while you were growing, learned preference (all those years in ballet or practicing sports "ready" position), and then there's the way that these preferences create forces when you walk, which really cements the position into the body. Your bones and muscles have adapted to decades of your habitual loading, so standing with your feet aligned properly will feel weird. Do it anyway.

## STEP 2: FEET PELVIS WIDTH

Get your ankles the width of your pelvis. The bony protrusions on the right and left side of your pelvis (commonly referred to as your hip bones) should be directly over the center of your ankles.

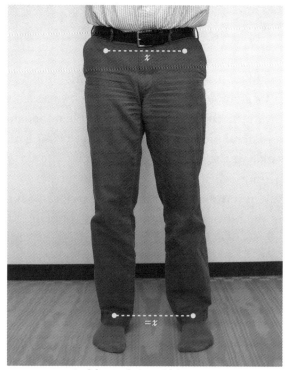

Ankles pelvis-width apart

Why? If your feet are closer together (more likely if you're a woman) or farther apart (more likely if you're a man) then you're creating particular loads to the knees that are associated with knee degeneration. Keeping your ankles at the correct width allows you to hold yourself up with the major muscle groups that do this job the best, rather than relying on passive structures like your ligaments. Also, in order to (eventually) walk in better alignment, you need your feet to be pelvis-width apart to engage both the lateral hip and butt musculature needed to walk with good posterior push-off (discussed in the section on treadmills).

## STEP 3: LEGS VERTICAL

Your pelvis (containing your center of mass while standing) should be back over your heels, instead of out over the front of your foot. When looking at yourself from the side (your profile), your hip joint, knee joint, and ankle joint should all stack vertically.

Why? For starters, the soft tissues in the middle of your foot (hello, plantar fascia!) don't bear your weight as well as the giant heel bone in your rear foot. But for the main course: Standing with your pelvis out in front of your foot puts unnecessary loads on your quadriceps and psoas, which in

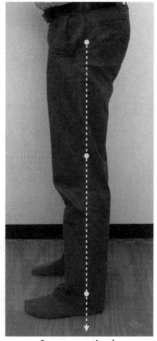

Legs vertical

turn messes with your knees. And all the weight you work to carry on the front of your body is weight you're not working to carry on your backside. If you're wondering where your butt muscle has gone, check out how much time you spend with your pelvis out in front of you. Share the love, and give your butt something to work against all day long. Let's give "Office Butt" a new meaning, shall we? Back those hips up, baby.

## STEP 4: PELVIS NEUTRAL

The pelvis is made up of the Anterior Superior Iliac Spines (ASIS), which are the most prominent anterior (front) superior (above) bony projections on the right and left side of your pelvis. People often refer to these points as the hipbones (as in, "Put your hands on your hips"). The pubic symphysis (PS) is the joint at which the two hipbones come together. It is the lowest bony prominence before your pelvis wraps around to the under-carriage.

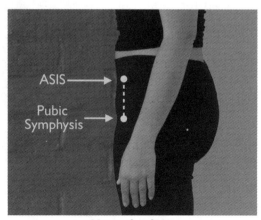

Neutral pelvis

Align your ASIS and PS vertically. Why? Your pelvis sets the stage for your spine. In the same way that a vase cannot sit "right" on a tilted table, your spine cannot sit optimally, relative to the gravitational force, unless your pelvis allows it to do so. Alignment of the pelvis is super important when you're standing all day long because the integrity of your spine (vertebrae, discs, and spinal ligaments) depends on it. The tilt of your pelvis also affects the muscles that attach to it. Of most importance when you're on your feet are the muscles of the abdomen. In order to keep your trunk muscles firing, they have to be at a length that optimizes their ability to generate force.

Quick explanation: A muscle is made of tiny components called sarcomeres. A muscle only moves because these sarcomeres have overlapping parts that provide the ability to shorten or lengthen. Your habitual positioning changes the amount these sarcomeres overlap—or don't—which in turn changes the leverage between the parts of sarcomere and thus within the muscle itself. Again, for a deeper explanation, read *Move Your DNA*.

Excessive tucking of the pelvis (or untucking—also a problem) reduces the intra-muscular leverage and therefore the stability of the spine when maintaining a single position over time. Of course, you'll want to be moving your pelvis (and whole body, for that matter) throughout the day, but in general, when you're in place, maintaining a neutral pelvis means you're allowing your low back to maintain the appropriate amount of curve for your particular stature (as long as you're also following step 5), which means much less back pain.

## STEP 5: RIBS DOWN

After aligning your pelvis, put your hands on your waist.
Now, slide your hands up so they encircle your ribcage. With
each hand, feel for the lowest part of your rib in the front of
your body, and drop those protrusions (each side being its
own "point") until the front part of the lowest rib is stacked
vertically over the front of the pelvis. Your ribs should sink
right into your abdominal flesh.

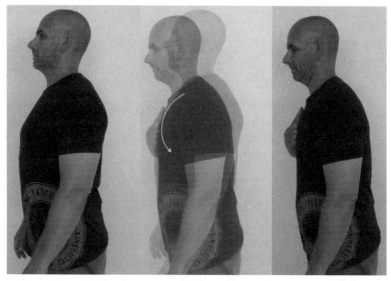

Lower your ribs to neutral

Why? Your spine is connected to your ribs. When you
thrust and/or lift your chest you're bringing your spine along
for the ride. Which means that you can't have a neutral
spine without first having a neutral ribcage. When you lift
and jut out your chest (which, I know, is often given as a
misguided tip for better posture), you're actually shearing

some vertebrae in your lower back and forcing the vertebrae in your neck to adjust unnaturally as well. Lowering your ribs also adjusts the fiber length of your diaphragm, allowing for better breathing. This alignment marker in particular exposes some unpleasant truths about the actual curve of your spine—especially the extra-curved upper back that almost all of us mask with our constant rib thrusting. Don't fret. Getting rid of the mask exposes where to focus your stretching and instantly alleviates undesirable loads on the spine. Even if your posture (how something looks) doesn't appear as good with your ribs down, your alignment (how something works) is better for the adjustment. You know that period of time when you started a new activity—maybe running—and you looked all flushed and red, arms and legs kind of wonky? But with training, adaptations came and soon you were doing that same activity, only looking much more awesome. Postural adjustments are like this as well. As you actively call on new positioning, the muscles from the top of your head to the bottom of your feet start to support you in a subtle, yet constant way. With time comes additional muscle mass specific to generate the forces associated with holding your body in a more symmetrical (read: well-balanced) way, eventually allowing you to relax and be supported in an outstanding-looking posture.

## STEP 6: KNEE PITS NEUTRAL

Stand with legs bare, feet straight, and your back to a mirror; turn around to look at the back of your knees and you will see four lines (two on each leg) that mark the tendons of your hamstring muscles. Ideally all four of these should align directly behind you, as your feet point straight ahead.

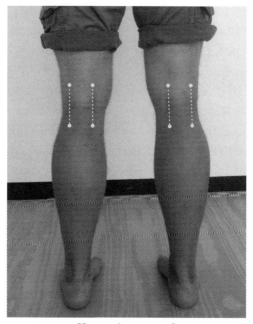

Knee pits neutral

This means that your ankles and knees can best hinge in the direction you are walking, which is typically forward. Unfortunately, in most cases, these hamstring tendons don't line up (for reasons similar to why your feet tend to drift out over time). To get those hammies straight, most people will need to externally rotate (rotate the front of the thighs away from each other). Watch in the mirror, rotating until you've brought all four lines to a neutral position. Please note that it's unlikely that your right and left leg will be rotating the same amount. The turnout of our feet is rarely symmetrical, which means the correction won't be either. When you are first starting to align your feet and then your knees, it's almost impossible to keep the sole of the foot in contact with the ground. Ideally your feet would be much more mobile—wearing shoes has clumped all the joints of the mid-foot together. This is why the cobblestone mat I'll discuss in a bit can really help out your whole body. For now, don't force your feet to stay down when externally rotating your thighs. Let the inner edges of the feet come up. They'll need to less over time if you're working on mobilizing your foot!

Why are you doing this? As I'll flesh out later on, standing injuries are common to the lower leg. Collapsed standing, what I call a "schmeared" ankle, occurs when your thighs roll in toward each other, taking the ankle in and down with them. The blood vessels inside your legs depend on active muscle engagement to maintain the geometry and suppleness of the arteries and veins. To stand sloppily is not only to tax your musculoskeletal system, but also to overburden the cardiovascular system within those muscles. Your lower leg is particularly at risk because it is under your weight all day long. The least you can do is to consciously support the athletic endeavor of standing in an aligned and symmetrical manner the entire time you are upright.

## STEP 7: KNEE CAP RELEASE

The position of your knee caps is not fixed, and is subject to the muscular tension pattern of your thigh muscles. Balanced standing (that is, where all muscles are encouraged to participate) doesn't require constant tension in the front of the thigh. Hence, if your patellas (knee caps) are locked into a "pulled upward" position, then your quads are doing too much of the work. Drop them by anchoring your weight back into your heels (which is where it should be anyway), thereby turning off the gripping motion of the quads.

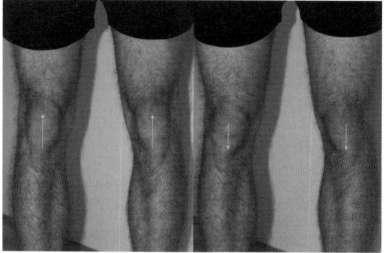

Relax the knee caps

Why? "Locked" knees is a leg position that subjects the body to blood-flow altering configurations—either hyperextension (when your knee joint is behind the vertical line established by your hip and ankle) or constant tension of the quadriceps muscles. Just as your band teacher or military sergeant might have warned you, locking your knees all day long is one way to reduce necessary blood flow. If you're going to try and spend more time upright during the day in the name of health, you'll want to make sure that you stand well, so that all of you is healthier for it.

## STEP 8: HEAD RAMPED UP

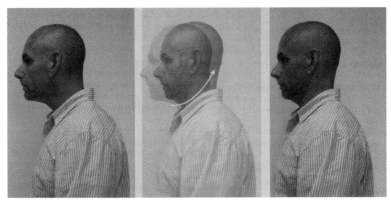

Ramp up the head

Once your ribcage is in a neutral position, slide your head back toward the wall behind you until your ears stack up over your shoulder. Don't pick your head up by the chin, and don't lift your chest (read: ribcage) to achieve this position. Each of these efforts is created by a lot of movement about a *single* hinge in the neck or back, which is not a good idea. Better, let the ramping motion be created by the efficient interaction of *many* joints. When you're looking to fix the curvature of your spine—anywhere between your head and pelvis—it is helpful to remember that curves are created by the actions of many parts. Ramping is a twofer. It not only helps to restore the neutral curve in the neck but also alleviates the excessive curvature in the upper back (for even mo' betta breathing, better back loading, less shoulder impingement)—a problem you may have only discovered once you aligned your ribs correctly.

**RESEARCH CORNER**

While your head weighs the same no matter its position, the amount its weight deforms the structures it connects to is influenced by where it sits. The more forward the head is to the spine, and the more the head nods forward (think how you position your head to read the screen of your smart phone or, gasp!, this book), the greater the load to the upper spine. Take-away: Ramp it up! (See page 55 for a simple head position adjustment.)

Hansraj, K.K. (2014). Assessment of Stresses in the Cervical Spine Caused by Posture and the Position of the Head. *Surgical Technology International, 25,* 277-279.

## STANDING ALL DAY IN SHOES

Now that I've given you all the objective markers to ensure you're in a neutral position, hear this: *There is no way to stand in neutral while wearing positive-heeled shoes.* Please note that the term "positive-heeled" does not refer to a heel being "good," but rather any shoe with a heel raised higher off the ground than the toes.

Many associate the term "heel" with a woman's dress shoe, but almost all shoes—men's and athletic shoes included—have a moderate to significant rise to them. The elevated heel found in most footwear takes many joints out of their neutral alignment (limiting potential ranges of motion) as well as relocates your center of mass away from your heels (where it should be) and onto the balls of your feet. This means that many of the benefits of standing and doing your exercises (coming next) will be negated by tissue loads created by wearing shoes.

The trouble with elevated heel shoes is that in order to

wear them, your bones and muscles have to move from
neutral. To the non-biomechanical eye, it might look like
someone is standing up just fine, but upon further investiga-
tion, the axes of the entire body adjust and are "off " when
you're wearing a positive-heeled shoe.

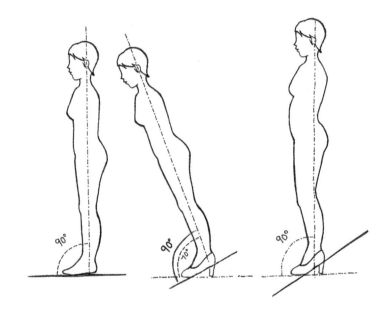

I'm not talking about the extremes of a stiletto here, but
actually any mildly elevated shoe, such as a typical running
shoe, leisure shoe, or men's dress shoe (pictured on next
page).

If you dress up for the office in elevated heel shoes, the
amount of time you spend sitting has probably saved your
feet from trouble! So, before you jump up and hike your
keyboard up to your standing *in heels* desk height, take a

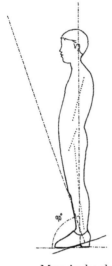

Man in heels

moment to understand the footwear issue and make a plan to mitigate the damage created by standing in elevated heels.

Heels move your center of mass and your center of pressure (COP) from the back of the foot to the front—where the tiny, delicate bone, tendon, and ligament structures are simply ill-equipped to adapt to this unnatural load. This forward shift in your COP is an injury waiting to happen. If you've ever checked out the skeletal formation of the foot, think about getting your weight back over the incredibly dense heel bone and away from the more delicate and dynamic structure of the mid-foot area. Using your entire foot while walking is great, but standing in place for a long time (not natural) in shoes that move your center of mass excessively forward (also not natural) makes it hard to use an ancestral-health or a physiological argument to support standing over sitting. So, to stay out of your favorite podiatrist's office, you've got to transition out of traditional elevated heel shoes and into something more healthy. Fortunately, the minimalist shoe movement is booming these days, and there are numerous office-appropriate options to choose from while still looking legit in a buttoned-up workplace. Invest in some professional-yet-minimal footwear, and/or keep a pair of totally flat shoes at your desk and discreetly switch out of your clunkers into a shoe with little to no elevation of the heel when you are standing up at your desk. I hate to be the bearer (and especially the reiterator!) of bad news, but there is simply no way to stand with good alignment (remember, alignment is about forces and not how hot you look) if you are wearing elevated heel shoes. Think about it. Stacking enthusiastic standup desk efforts on top of weak, mal-aligned feet is no different from trying to build a structurally sound house on the bank of an eroding river. Pan out and look at the big picture; this isn't about short-term success but optimal, long-term tissue adaptation.

## ANATOMY BIT

There is nothing that makes me cringe more than seeing an ad for a standing workstation featuring a woman in stilettos. Seriously? Doctors don't even recommend that you walk around in those killers, so imagine the damage you can do to the bones, muscles, and connective tissues in the feet by standing in high heels all day long!

### WHEN STANDING HURTS YOUR BACK, RE-CHECK YOUR RIBS

A common cause of back pain, especially when standing, is the rib thrust. Sometimes you do this because you were told to keep your chest up, and sometimes this position is created by excessive tension in your psoas muscle. No matter how your thrust came to be, take this test to see if you are a habitual rib-thruster.

Stand with your heels three to four inches from a wall. Keeping your butt touching but not overly pressing into the wall, straighten the legs until they're vertical, as in step 3. Next, bring your shoulders, arms,

## WHEN STANDING HURTS YOUR BACK... (CONT'D)

and back of the head against the wall. You should have a small space underneath your waist where your low back naturally curves in, but your middle back (the ribs/bra-strap/heart-rate-monitor area) should also be touching the wall.

If your waist is entirely on the wall, you are overly tucking your pelvis under. Adjust this by tilting your tailbone out toward the wall until your pelvis is in neutral, as in step 4. Once the space reappears, try to get your mid-back, shoulders, and head against the wall *without straining*.

If your parts don't easily line up on this simple test, then it's likely that the upper part of your spine has lost its mobility.

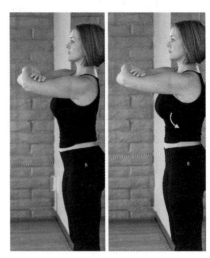

Ribs against a wall before/after

Ideally, each of the upper back's vertebrae should move a little to get back toward the wall. But with the loss of vertebral mobility it is common to get the upper hunk of the spine back to the wall by moving the ribcage as a single unit—sliding the entire chest area forward, thus creating compression and ligament strain in the lumbar spine. Pain in the lower back when standing is often created by this excessive pressure on the vertebral discs.

To decrease the pain, drop your ribs regularly. As for corrective exercises, shoulder-opening exercises done without shearing the ribs (i.e., maintaining "ribs down") can also improve the mobility of this area. See the thoracic and nerve stretch in Chapter 7.

chapter 6

# WORKING OUT ON COMPANY TIME: THE SUBTLE STUFF

MOST OF US understand "movement" to mean large physical feats or sweaty bouts of exercise. While large movements and sensible workout routines are great, the smaller, more subtle movements that you engage in without a second thought throughout the day are just as important to your health. Smaller movements—like the rotation of your ribs, the work down the outer thigh as you stand on one foot, and the ongoing, isometric contraction of the calf muscles as they hold your body upright—all serve a purpose when it comes to maintaining healthy biological function.

And while it's tough to sprint and work at the same time,

you can totally get away with all sorts of health-improving smaller movements without attracting much attention or leaving the confines of your workspace.

Following are five exercises that, when done simultaneously with aligning your points, keep your body "moving" when you're just standing there.

## GASTROC CALF STRETCH

Place a thick folded and rolled towel (or a rolled yoga mat or a half foam roller) on the floor in front of you by your work-station. Step onto the towel with a bare or minimally shod foot, placing the ball of the foot on the top of the towel and keeping your heel on the floor.

Adjust the foot so that it points straight forward, and keep your stretching leg straight at all times.

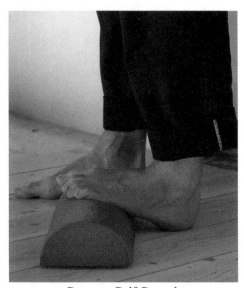

Gastroc Calf Stretch

Keeping your body upright (shoulders and hips over heels; mind those alignment markers), step forward with the opposite foot.

The tighter the lower leg muscles and tendons, the harder it will be to bring the other foot in front. You might even have to keep the non-stretching leg behind the towel. Some people can bring the opposite foot forward only with lots of butt, quad, and jaw clenching—only step as far forward as you can while keeping everything else relaxed. Repeat other side.

By doing this stretch, you're not only working to undo decades of positive-heel-wearing and chair-sitting, you're also improving the amount of work done by the skeletal pump on your venous return system when you're moving. You simply can't do this exercise too much! There are days when I Gastroc Calf Stretch one leg, and then the other, *the entire time* I'm standing at my desk!

## SOLEUS CALF STRETCH

The Gastroc Calf Stretch targets the gastrocnemius muscle of the calf group by keeping the knee from bending. But there is another muscle in the calf group, called the soleus, that is better stretched

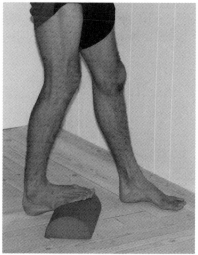

Soleus Calf Stretch

when the ankle joint gets even smaller (increased dorsiflexion), which requires a bent knee. Standing on the towel (or mat or half foam roller) with the ball of one foot up on the dome and its heel on the ground, bend the same leg's knee—pushing it slightly forward—as you press that same heel toward the ground.

### IT'S NOT *ONLY* THE SHOES

Calf tension doesn't only stem from how your shoes fix your ankle into a slight toe point, but also from how a chair "casts" your knee at 90°. If you're after more mobile calves, you should also reduce the amount of time you spend with your knees bent—a position that also shortens the posterior leg muscles. If you've gone out of your way to avoid heeled shoes for foot or lower leg pain, consider this: Sitting in a chair requires your gastrocnemius (the largest of the calf muscles) to shorten more than wearing heels does. Sitting while wearing heels? Well, that's just a double whammy.

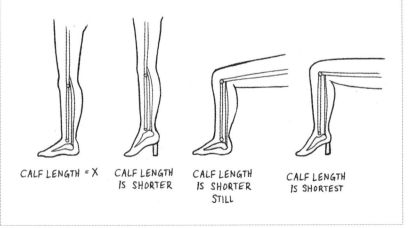

CALF LENGTH = X     CALF LENGTH IS SHORTER     CALF LENGTH IS SHORTER STILL     CALF LENGTH IS SHORTEST

## WEIGHT-SHIFTING

Standing in body "neutral" position, except with feet slightly wider, shift your weight so you're standing on only your left leg. Be especially careful to untuck your pelvis and back your hips up. Try doing this without bending either knee at all—just slowly press your left foot into the floor, focusing on using the muscles around the outside of your left hip to push you to the right. Next, try with the right leg, calling on those muscles to push you back to the left. Then, see if you can get your non-weight-bearing hip into the air *without using your waist muscles at all*—just by pressing your standing leg farther into the floor. You can shift your weight like this anytime you're standing around "doing nothing"—no equipment required!

## FOOT EXERCISES

Here are some interesting stats. You've got 26 bones, 33 joints, and over 100 muscles, tendons, and ligaments in each foot. And how much do you work those muscles? Hardly at all. Modern footwear and the constant flat and level surfaces we walk upon have resulted in a casting of these joints for most of our waking hours, and we've got the muscle atrophy to prove it.

Your feet can really take a beating after standing on the floor hours and hours at a time, which is why you've got to move these tiny parts to offset the static loading.

Standing in alignment, weight back in your heels (this is crucial), spread all of your toes away from each other without letting them lift away from the ground.

Right now, you might not have any mobility in some of

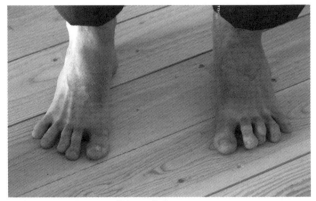

Spread the toes

your toes—just keep working on these tiny muscles and eventually they will wake up.

Now, while standing in alignment, lift your big toe while keeping all the other toes down. Keep your big toe pointing straight ahead; don't let it deviate laterally (towards your other toes).

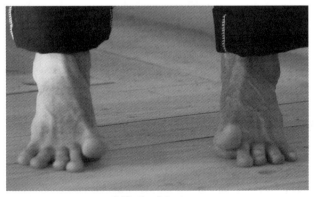

Lift the big toes

Make sure you're keeping the ball of your foot in contact with the floor—it's common to cheat by rolling onto the sides of your foot. Once you've lifted the big toe, move to the second toe on each foot. Then the third. Then the fourth. And the baby toe too. Lift each one individually, and put them back down one at a time. Yep, pretty darn difficult. Actually, it can take years to restore good muscle separation and mobility to your toes, but even making a decent effort on a regular basis will stimulate that musculature again.

You can also purchase a cobblestone (or cobblestone-ish) mat to stand on in between other stretches. It's fairly impossible to move the intrinsic muscles (smaller muscles within the foot) on your own—were you in nature these muscles would have been moved for you via the ever-changing shape of the natural terrain humans once walked upon. When you can't make it, fake it. Stone mats have a rough surface simulating a natural stone bed, giving your feet a necessary workout.

Interestingly, one study on cobblestone mats demonstrated that those doing walking exercise on a cobble mat experienced greater decreases in blood pressure than those just walking over flat ground.

For many this supports a belief in the merits of acupressure or reflexology in the feet, but perhaps a more direct explanation is the effect mobile joints and working muscles have on the volume of blood within the arteries of the lower extremities. More working parts—even smallish parts in the feet—mean more blood in the capillaries and less blood within the larger vessels of the arteries (where blood pressure is measured). For me, standing on a cobblestone mat while at my desk is a subtle way to work the intrinsic muscles of my feet—keeping me moving, even when the bulk of my body is standing still. Clever, I know.

## ABOUT YOUR EYES

The habit of sitting all day wreaks havoc on more than the obvious structures like the heart or thigh muscles. In the same way your legs are (semi)-permanently casted into hip and knee flexion by a chair, your eyes are casted and thereby weakened when they are engaged for hours staring at a screen a fixed distance away.

Your eyes have muscles too. Just as doing a million bicep curls and nothing else with your arms would result in a very particular arm shape (and proclivity for injury), our eyes have been utilized in one repetitive way (i.e., always 20 inches away from the screen), making them great in one way and weak in all the others. Strength that resides next to weakness within a structure makes that structure ripe for degeneration, so let's talk about cross-training your eyes.

Just as the angle between your upper and lower arm correlates with a specific shortness of the biceps muscle group, the distance between your eye and what you're looking at constitutes a specific shortness in the eye's ciliary muscles (responsible for helping the lens change shape to focus on different objects). If you were to put your arm in a cast, eventually the biceps muscles would permanently shorten. You would then have great difficulty just straightening your arm out!

The same goes for your eyes. When you engage in *repetitive looking* (I think I might have just coined a new term here) for hours upon hours with little to no break, your eye muscles atrophy to the extent that they become less able to focus on objects of disparate lengths or quickly transition between focusing at different distances.

So, here's what you need to do to keep your eyes from plateauing: First, notice when your face gets way close to the computer. You know, when you're all deep into your work and your body is collapsing toward whatever you're working on? Knock that off and back yourself up. Keep yourself as far away from the screen as your head ramping (alignment step 8) and arm length will allow. Note that a keyboard that is separate from your computer will allow you to back up even more. As long as you're not straining (read: clenching your eyes) to read the screen, backing up is a good thing. But really, backing up these few inches—while helpful—won't get you the eye-relaxing effect you're after. To really give your eyes a break and keep their muscles supple, you must take your eyes away from your computer and look at the farthest point away from you. Ideally you should be able to look out a window, where the farthest object is hundreds of feet away—the cross-training equivalent of running if you are typically a swimmer. If there is no window, then look across the room, hopefully into a different office, which gets you about 30 feet worth of eye relation. More like cross-training with a leg press machine when you're used to cycling every day. Take "look beyond your computer" breaks during your workday, at least a quick glance every five minutes, and more extended gazes every 30 minutes. There are also software programs available that can act as a personal trainer to your eyes and dim your screen at a pre-determined frequency and length of time. Keep your eyes healthy. Seeing clearly is one of those functions we take for granted until it starts to go!

## YOUR SUBTLE MOVEMENT EXERCISE RX

The subtle movements I've discussed don't follow a "do this X amount of times, Y times a day" format. Each of these movements can be done the entire time you are working. Obviously, an exception is the distance eye-gazing, which would make working on your computer difficult if you were looking away all day long. The more you can think "alignment" and the more you constantly work your body even while staying at your desk, the better the transition out of your chair will be for you.

# chapter 7

# BIG MOVEMENTS TO DO AT YOUR DESK

THE FOLLOWING ARE exercises that will probably require that you take a work break. Utilizing three- to five-minute exercise breaks throughout the day, you can either practice just one per break, or you can flow through all of them in one movement period. The results are entirely different and both are beneficial in their own way. I suggest that on some days you work on each individual exercise to reach a deeper level in one area. On other days, flow through all of them, on every break, to mobilize more of you more often.

## THORACIC STRETCH

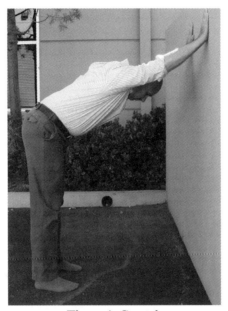

Thoracic Stretch

Place your hands on your desk or the wall. Keeping your hands touching, walk backward, dropping your chest toward the ground. Keeping your feet straight, back your pelvis up until your hips are behind your ankles, legs are straight (quads relaxed), and your tailbone lifted. Make sure you're not thrusting your ribs. For an added bonus, turn your palms and "elbow pits" (the inside of your arm, opposite to the bony elbow) up. This is a great way to gently load the tension in the shoulder joints and de-mouse your arms!

## DOUBLE CALF STRETCH

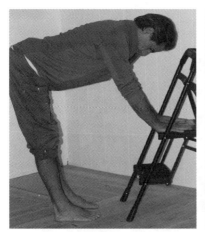
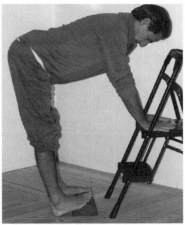

Double Calf Stretch          Double Calf Stretch with dome

This move places a great load on the tissues that keep your pelvis in a tucked position. Place your hands on the seat of your chair or on your desk. Line up the outside edges of your feet and straighten your legs all the way (quads relaxed). Back your hips up behind your heels and make sure all your toes are liftable. Keeping your knees from bending and your ribs from thrusting, untuck your pelvis until you feel the muscles down the back of the leg. To intensify this stretch, externally rotate your thighs to neutral (alignment step 6) during this exercise to bring even more of your thigh muscle fibers into the stretch. Want even more? Place the front of both feet up on a half foam roller or rolled towel.

## WALL ANGELS

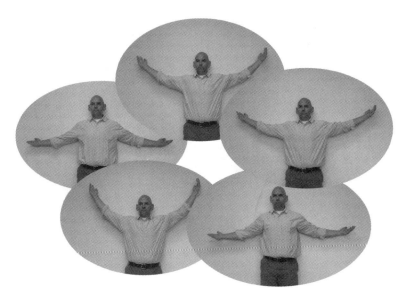

Wall Angels

Stand with your back against a wall, your feet about three to four inches away. Bring your hips and ribcage back until they touch the wall; this will keep you from thrusting your ribcage. Reach your arms out to the side, making a T, with your palms facing out (not toward the wall). Slowly, keeping the backs of the hands and wrists against the wall, work your arms overhead, stopping once the arms or the ribs pull away from the wall. Repeat in a smooth fashion, like you're making snow angels on the wall.

## SEATED AND STANDING PIRIFORMIS STRETCH

As you might have guessed, this stretch targets your piriformis, a muscle deep in your hip that connects your sacrum
to the top of the thigh bone. When this puppy is stiff your
hips can't articulate well, the motion of the leg places inappropriate tension on the sacroiliac (SI) joint, and it can also
irritate the heck out of the sciatic nerve. Sitting on the edge
of a chair, keep your left foot on the floor and cross your
right leg over so the ankle is resting on the left knee. Untuck
your pelvis—follow the protocol outlined for better sitting
on page 38—and then slowly lean forward. It doesn't take
much leaning to feel a deep stretch in the piriformis.

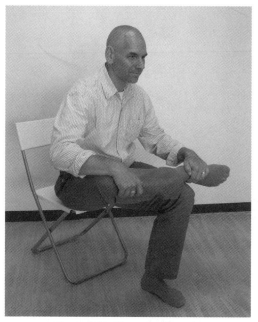

Seated Piriformis Stretch

For an additional challenge, do this stretch while standing. Using your desk for balance, hook the ankle of one leg over the knee of the other, then lower your hips toward the ground—no, it's not going to be much—while keeping your standing leg's knee directly above the ankle.

You'll not only get the stretch in one hip, you'll be working the muscles of the other leg and your trunk to participate in holding you up. Time-maximizer, for sure.

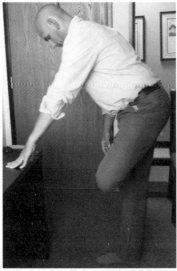
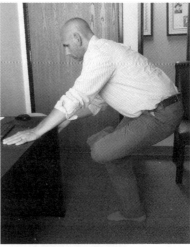

Standing Piriformis Stretch, getting ready

Standing Piriformis Stretch, sitting back

## PELVIC SLIDE

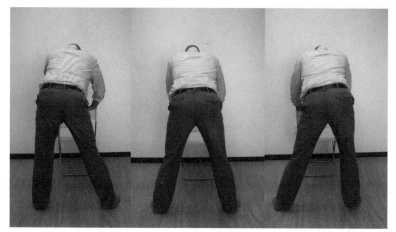

Pelvic Slide

Stand with your legs more than hip-width apart, feet pointing forward, with a chair or desk in front of you. Bend forward until your hands are resting on the seat of the chair (or arms on a desk), and relax your pelvis and spine toward the ground (try not to let your back arch like a cat's). Back up your hips until they are behind your heels (you'll feel your hamstrings start to stretch), and then shift your pelvis toward the right leg and then toward the left, without migrating forward. Imagine both butt cheeks are on a wall, which will keep one hip from hiking (i.e., one side of your waist from shortening); the only motion should be the pelvis gliding over the tops of the thighs. You can play with different widths of your feet—the wider you go, the more it will change the stretch.

## NERVE STRETCH

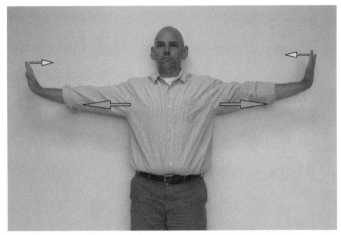

Nerve Stretch

Begin by reaching your hands away from you, making a T and a "STOP! In the name of love" motion of the hand. Spreading the fingers away from each other, slowly work your fingertips back toward the main axis of your body. Keep your middle fingers pointing up, your thumbs pointing forward, and your elbow pits facing the ceiling. To intensify the sensation, don't think of pushing your hands away from you (which just straightens the elbow) but of reaching the entire arm bone away from you—like your shoulder is in traction. Hello! You should feel a sensation running down both arms. Yes, nerves, like muscles, can stretch, but really what you're doing is just moving your arms through ranges not created by the work environment. By doing so, you keep all your parts—nerves included—gliding smoothly around each other (read: adhesion-free).

# THE WAITER

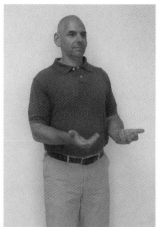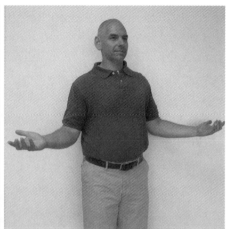

The Waiter

Standing, bend your elbows to 90°, with your palms up (like you're holding a tray in your hands). Keeping your hands up and your elbows bent, slowly move your hands laterally (away from your imaginary midline) until your right hand is off to the right and your left to the left. Bring them back together. Initially you can do this *sans* equipment, but for even more work, do this motion using light-resistance exercise tubing or a set of hand weights (no more than five pounds). This is a great way to introduce external rotation to the shoulder, especially following hours of the internal rotation necessary for keyboarding. A keyboard that splits is one way to reduce the amount of time spent in internal rotation, as is using your keyboard less. Voice dictation software can allow you to work without using your hands and shoulders, allowing you to "waiter" while you work.

## COBBLESTONE MAT WALKING

Normally I'd say that all walk breaks should go down away from your computer and out of your office but sometimes the opportunity arises for you to walk (i.e., be away from your computer) while you're still working—like when you take a call. In this case, use a cobblestone mat for more than just standing on, and instead of just taking the call, log in some steps with the added benefit of foot and ankle mobilization.

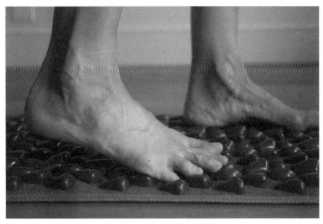

Cobblestone mat walking

# chapter 8

# STANDING AND INJURY

I WOULDN'T PRESUME to know all the reasons human resource departments the world over are reluctant to move everyone out of their chairs and into standing workstations. However, I have a couple of reasons of my own as to why this might not be the best idea.

No matter how much I present the underlying tenets of physiology (it takes time to adapt, for example) and a plan for progressing without creating tissue damage, the super-motivated often skim over that part with an I TOTALLY GOT THIS attitude and jump right to the part where they click on the purchase button for the new stand-up-all-day desk.

If you have any friends who are teachers—another profession that stands a lot, at least nine months out of the year—talk to them about how it feels those first few weeks back at school after being on summer break. It's painful or fatiguing, or both. And most teachers can sit down quite a bit throughout the day—at least more than you can

MANY SUPER-MOTIVATED FOLKS JUMP RIGHT INTO A NEW STAND-UP-ALL-DAY DESK WITHOUT CONSIDERING THE BEST PLAN TO VARY THE WORKPLACE ENVIRONMENT AND MINIMIZE TISSUE DAMAGE.

if you totally eradicate all other options besides STAND.

Smart transitioning has less to do with standing being a good or bad idea, and more to do with your body needing time to get used to long bouts of standing in order to correctly recruit muscles and utilize them well. If your HR department has concerns about your strength or personal level of health as you aspire to integrate standup time at work, share your training program plan with them. They're much more likely to sign off on your new office design if you let them know you are aware of potential issues and are taking measures to mitigate "dangers" they may perceive as being directly related to your new office that *they've* installed (easing their fears about being liable for your standup desk injury, you see?).

Another reason I hesitate to present standing workstations as the best solution has to do with standing injuries. And yes, there are injuries associated with prolonged standing!

**TRANSITIONING APPROPRIATELY**

A fairly accomplished runner can complete a marathon run (26.2 miles) in around four hours. That's four hours *less* than the not-as-vigorous-but-still-physiologically-taxing event of standing a full workday at your desk. I'll bet that, after spending a few years on the couch, you wouldn't stroll down to the registration tent of your local 26.2 mile race and jump onto the starting line. If you did, you'd be likely to fail, because your tissues would not be up to the task. Your tissues would not be strong enough to assume the loads created by running or walking this distance or for this duration. People pulled randomly out of the crowd would break down after anywhere from a few miles to perhaps halfway through. It's obvious that a daunting physical effort like a marathon requires a sincere commitment to training for many months if not years. Through diligent and sensible training, you incrementally increase your loads over time to allow your cells to adapt.

Standing workstations are no different in that they require endurance and musculoskeletal strengths you probably don't yet have. To maximize the whole-body benefits of getting out of your chair, recognize you've got to gradually increase your standing intervals over time, and also dedicate portions of the day to doing transitioning exercises.

One of the points lost on many is that our collective movement into chairs was brought about by the injuries, to the low back and feet for example, that arose in populations that stood all day.

Musculoskeletal issues like knee and back pain that come from sitting can be mitigated by smart progression and changing *how* you stand—which is why alignment while

## ANATOMY BIT

Varicose veins (*varix* is Latin, for spread—stretch, separate—apart; *-ose* is also Latin, for "full of") are veins that have become enlarged and twisted. They can occur anywhere, but are most common in the lower leg and groin. They are benign in most cases (although sometimes painful). Avoiding further damage to venous tissues can prevent complications that arise from long-term decreases in circulation common to varicosity.

standing at work is critical. By minding your alignment points, you've really got that one covered. But perhaps the most prevalent health issue associated with standing—varicose veins— is *not* offset by how you stand. It's being upright *and still* that contributes to this issue.

Varicose veins are not just a throwback to the days of standing on the line at a factory. Jobs like clerking at a department store and nursing are still commonly associated with vein problems in the lower leg and groin.

Allow me to present the most basic lecture ever on the inner workings of your venous return system: When your blood leaves your heart, it flows through the arterial system (those red lines in an anatomy book) with the assistance of your heart and skeletal muscle. Once blood has reached its final destination (whatever capillary it went to), it returns via your venous system (normally drawn as blue lines). Unlike the arterial system, the venous system can't capitalize on the work performed by the heart, so veins rely on additional mechanisms to avoid blood pooling while making the long and upward (read: against gravity) trek back to the lungs, where the blood becomes re-oxygenated and the cycle starts over. These "additional mechanisms" include the pumping action of muscle (muscles contracting and releasing when you're moving around) as well as specialized valves. These valves sort of help your blood "climb up" your veins; after opening to let blood up toward the head, they snap shut behind (read: underneath) the volume of blood that just moved toward the lungs. Like salmon swimming upstream, compartments of blood "stair-step" up your veins using the flap as a place to rest.

For a long time, varicose veins were believed to be a problem with the valves, but more recent research shows that the internal environment of a vein can cause a local change in the vein wall's genetic expression. For example, elevated stress hormones in the bloodstream, turbulent blood flow due to poor musculoskeletal alignment, or poor oxygen delivery to tissues (due to lack of movement, among other things) can leave a vein weakened and floppy. When you have a floppy venous wall, the valves no longer close off the vein and back-flow is allowed.

Couple a vein prone to back-flow with the higher pressures on the vein walls caused by standing and/or all-day stillness (with no more muscular pump helping the blood back up), and your veins will continue to progress down the varicose highway—not to mention the potential development of other issues like deep vein thrombosis, with which varicose veins have been associated. (I know I just said that varicosities are benign, but it's important to remember that these "benign" things that creep up in the body can be red flags for future ailments. They're your body's way of letting you know "something isn't right with your inner workings; please heed this signal.") When we couple injury-making forces with calves that *never* use their full range of motion because they have adapted to heeled shoes, when we sit the bulk of our life except to walk mostly on flat and level ground, the veins in the lower limb are primed for venous injury.

Keep the pressure down by loading and unloading your calves often. If you are already dealing with significant vein issues, the treadmill desk might be a better option than standing in place, so that you can keep your muscle pumps going all day long. If you're opting for well-aligned and constantly "moving" standing, then the two calf stretches described are your new best friends. In either case—walking or standing—excessive calf tension prevents the full use of your muscle pumps, so calf stretching is super important. If you add lots of foot work, wear zero-rise shoes, and take many movement breaks throughout the day, your circulatory system will thank you.

### ANTI-FATIGUE OR "SQUISHY" MATS

Most artificial surfaces have unnaturally low give to them, which means standing all day on concrete or other hard surfaces can be hard on the body. If your floor isn't carpeted, invest in a gel mat or other type of padded/comfort mat that reduces the loads to your body. Don't want to buy yet another thing? Fold over a yoga mat or towel a few times and you're good to go. Extra bonus: A slightly unstable mat ups the ante when it comes to your at-the-desk balance exercises!

**THE STANDING WORKSTATION CHECKLIST**

Pilots use checklists for every flight lest they forget some essential step to takeoff or landing. The following is not only a great way to cycle through your own body checks while at your workstation; it's also good information to share with your HR department about how you are assuming lots of responsibility when it comes to your workstation and your health.

1. Constantly monitor your alignment points (make a photocopy of page 97 and keep a low-profile copy taped to your monitor).

2. Use a half foam roller or rolled towel to stretch lower legs through the day for improved lower leg circulation.

3. Continuously shift your frame, using various, slightly different standing alignments to keep muscles active in a constantly changing way, also supporting the venous return system and minimizing tissue overload.

4. Sit or change positions when your muscles feel fatigued.

5. Take one- or two-minute movement breaks (e.g., walking short distances through the office) every 30 minutes. Go see someone in the flesh instead of calling or instant messaging them. Note: These are different from the three- to five-minute movement breaks specifically dedicated to corrective exercises.

6. Take one- to two-minute eye-breaks every 20 minutes.

chapter 9

# THE BIG PICTURE

I RECENTLY RECEIVED an email from one of my blog followers regarding his experience with the trend of alternative workstations:

*"About a couple years back, at my current job, the leadership team started plans to restructure the desk layout in the creative department. I lobbied aggressively for some standup influences, sending articles to my supervisor lauding the benefits of standup working. I soon became one of the first in our department to use a standing workstation, replete with a foam half-dome for calf-stretching! For a little while, I was called 'the hippie in*

*the corner' and got weird looks. However, fast forward to the present, and well more than half of our department is using them, and also are inclined to take frequent walking breaks. And guess what? The boost in productivity went through the roof! Your book on the diseases of modern living couldn't have come at a better time."*

It's exciting to see the problem of death-by-work being addressed, especially at a time when evidence has never been greater. But, rather than choosing to end this book with a "go forth with your health-making workstation" sentiment, I'd like to highlight that what we are attempting to do here is to fool Mother Nature by figuring out how to make eight hours spent in an office seem, to our bodies, like eight hours spent trekking through the Serengeti. Of course, that's not really what we're hoping for. We're simply trying to make it feel, to our body, less like eight hours in a tiny cage. Which is wonderful.

But you can only spend so much time (years) and money (thousands) trying to solve a problem (your job is costing you your health) before you notice that you haven't been working on the correct problem at all, and that in fact the problem is something you haven't yet acknowledged.

WE ARE ATTEMPTING TO FOOL MOTHER NATURE BY MAKING EIGHT HOURS SPENT IN AN OFFICE SEEM, TO OUR BODIES, LIKE EIGHT HOURS SPENT TREKKING THROUGH THE SERENGETI—OR AT LEAST LESS LIKE EIGHT HOURS SPENT IN A TINY CAGE!

When it comes to a tissue—bone, for example—beneficial adaptations to movement (like improved cross-sectional area or bone mineral density) are brought about by dynamic (continuously changing) loads, not static ones. Over time, bone—and all tissues, really—stops responding to routine loading signals.

This is why exercisers cross-train, right? To avoid plateauing and to challenge their bodies to experience performance breakthroughs. Well, what's happening now is that our health is literally plateauing—declining, really—at our desks, and the bar set by your desk isn't that high.

We're being radical here, but I'd like to suggest that we take it a step further and strive to restructure the workday entirely. And while we're at it, restructure the role of "work" itself in our lives.

The challenge to presenting material based on an evolutionary model's explanation of optimal health is to try and get these ancient principles to work in a modern setting. Yes, we need to work for a living, but who says that 10–50 percent of work can't be done from a home office, where we are free to stand barefoot and on cobblestone mats, do a sprint every 45 minutes in our driveway, or free ourselves from long commutes, tight belts, "business" shoes, and the stress and huge potential for distraction in the modern office? Who says that meetings have to be conducted in a boardroom and not while taking a group walk? Isn't oxygen crucial to problem solving?

In your world, are phone calls less professional when taken outside on a walk? If so, consider what would happen if both parties were walking. Immediate acceptance!

I, for one, do all of my phone calls—even important stuff

**RESEARCH CORNER**

**BRAINSTORMING GETS LEGS**

One study measured participants' creativity in four separate experiments in different settings: sitting, sitting outside, walking on a treadmill, and walking outside. Creative thinking was boosted during and immediately after walking, with walking outside producing the most novel and highest quality analogies.

Oppezzo, M. & Schwartz, D.L. (2014). Give Your Ideas Some Legs: The Positive Effect of Walking On Creative Thinking. *Journal of Experimental Psychology: Learning, Memory and Cognition, 40(4)*, 1142-1152.

like professional interviews and contract negotiations—while logging my daily miles. How about taking some inspiration from the progressive-minded Swedes, who are just now testing out potential increases in productivity and well-being brought about by a six-hour workday?

And it's not only that paid vacation norms in my country (United States) are miniscule compared to those of our friends in Europe, and many other nations across the globe. We seem to discount siestas and other built-in social customs promoting work/health balance. You can have the coolest, hippest, most progressive work environment ever, but if you spend too much time there—at the expense of family, friends, fitness, fun—then many of the intended benefits are inconsequential.

My point is, there are solutions, but in order to find them we have to make sure we are asking the right questions. A good question to start with is: Is your life's work working for you?

It is my hope that the answer, especially after reading and implementing the ideas in this book, is a resounding YES.

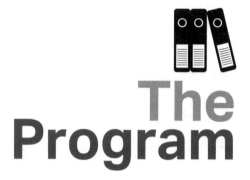

The
Program

## quick tips for a healthy, dynamic, well-aligned workplace

**MOVE**: There is no single best working position. Change positions frequently. Mix things up over the course of your day—sit, stand, stretch, move! Consider a variable keyboard.

**BREAK**: Take breaks for outdoor strolls as often as possible, or to just "hang out" on a monkey bar. Treadmill walking doesn't count!

**MELLOW OUT**: Minimize the amount of artificial light in your work environment. Strive to use natural light whenever possible. After dark, minimize artificial light and screen use.

**SIT WELL**: Take a seat, with your pelvis in neutral to promote optimal alignment from head to tail(bone). Sit on the edge of a chair, or use a stool, bench, kickstand device, or even a physio ball. No need for a fancy office chair to do the work. Use your muscles!

**STAND WELL**: Load your body efficiently. Begin with "feet forward," and work to keep the main long axis of your body stacked vertically. Pelvis neutral, not tucked! Ribs down, not forward. Knees neutral, thighs rotated, and head ramped! Wear minimalist shoes, or go barefoot if you can.

**STRETCH**: Stretch calves, work feet, shift weight. Stretch your eyes by focusing on distant objects every few minutes. Implement the big movements from Chapter 7 throughout the day.

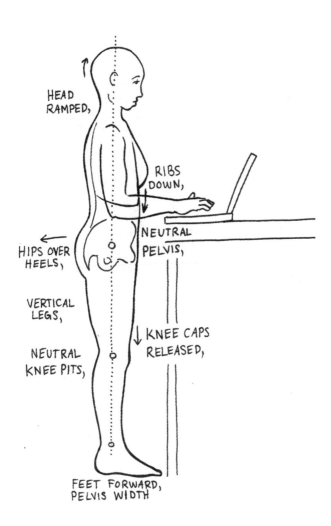

HEAD
RAMPED,

RIBS
DOWN,

NEUTRAL
PELVIS,

HIPS OVER
HEELS,

VERTICAL
LEGS,

↓ KNEE CAPS
RELEASED,

NEUTRAL
KNEE PITS,

FEET FORWARD,
PELVIS WIDTH

## exercises

### GASTROC CALF STRETCH

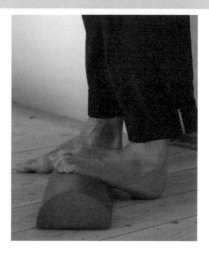

- Place the ball of your left foot on the apex of a half-foam roller or rolled-up folded towel, drop the heel all the way to the ground, and straighten that knee.
- Step forward with your right foot.
- If you can't bring your foot all the way forward, take a  smaller step.
- Keep your weight stacked vertically over the heel of whichever foot is farther back.
- Hold for a minute, then switch legs; do this three times each leg working up to a minute-long hold each time.

**ADVANCED VERSION:**
- Do this exercise while keeping your thighs in neutral (rotate your knee pits to neutral).

## SOLEUS CALF STRETCH

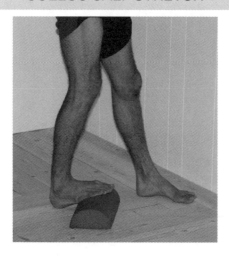

- After getting into Gastroc Calf Stretch position, bend the knees while keeping your heels down.
- Hold for up to a minute, then switch legs; repeat this as often as you do the Gastroc Calf Stretch.

**ADVANCED VERSION:**

- Do this exercise while keeping your thighs in neutral (rotate your knee pits to neutral).

## WEIGHT-SHIFTING

- Stand in body neutral, except with feet slightly wider.
- Shift your weight so you're standing on only your left leg.
- Keep pelvis in neutral and back your hips up.
- Without bending either knee, slowly press your left foot into the floor, using the muscles around the outside of your left hip to push you to the right.
- Do the same with the right leg.
- Raise your non-weight-bearing hip into the air without using your waist muscles at all, just pressing your standing leg farther into the floor.

## COBBLESTONE MAT WALKING

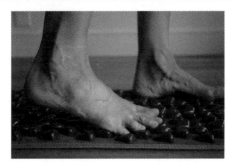

- When you can't take a walk outside, walk on a cobblestone mat during phone calls, quick meetings, brainstorming time.

## FOOT EXERCISES

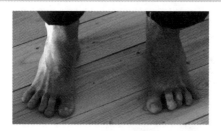

- Stand in body neutral, making sure to shift weight back toward your heels.
- Spread your toes away from each other without letting them lift away from the ground.

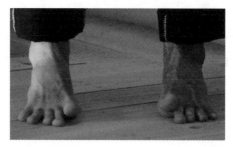

- Then lift your big toes while keeping all your other toes down.
- Keep your big toes pointing straight ahead; don't let them deviate laterally (toward their foot's pinkie toe).
- Keep the ball of your foot in contact with the floor.
- Once you've lifted the big toe, move to the second and then third, fourth, and fifth toes on each foot.
- Lift each one individually, and put them back down one at a time.
- You can also purchase a cobblestone mat to stand on in between other stretches.

## CROSS-TRAIN THE EYES

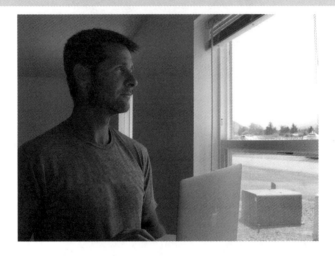

- Adjust the distance between your head and your monitor frequently.
- Look away from your computer and at the farthest point you can see (preferably out a window) for at least a quick glance every five minutes, and for an extended gaze every half hour.

## THORACIC STRETCH

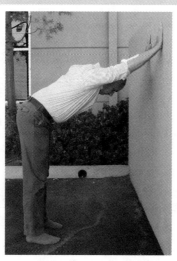

- Place your hands on your desk or the wall.
- Keeping your hands touching, walk backward, dropping your chest toward the ground.
- Keeping your feet straight, back your pelvis up until your hips are behind your ankles, legs are straight (quads relaxed), and your tail bone lifted. Don't thrust your ribs.
- Turn your palms and elbow pits up to gently load the tension in the shoulder joints.

## DOUBLE CALF STRETCH

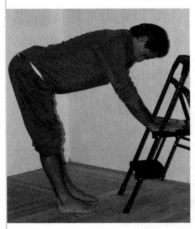 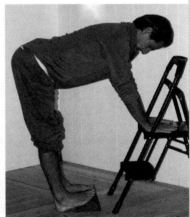

- Stand in front of a chair, facing the seat. With your feet pelvis-width apart, knees straight, and feet pointing forward, tip the pelvis forward until your palms rest on the chair.
- If you can't reach the chair without really bending the knees or rounding the back, make your seat height higher or move to a counter or desktop.
- Once your arms are down, see if you can allow your spine to drop down toward the floor, and your tailbone to lift toward the ceiling.
- Don't force your ribs to the floor or arch your back—just consciously relax the spine to the ground as much as you can.
- To intensify, place the balls of the feet on top of a half foam roller or rolled towel.
- Hold for up to a minute and repeat often throughout the day.

## WALL ANGELS

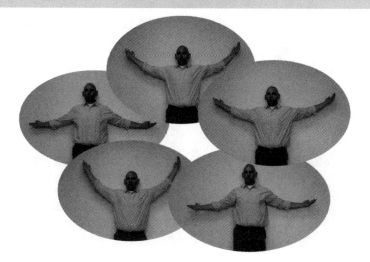

- Stand with your back against a wall, your feet about three to four inches away.
- Bring your hips and ribcage back until they touch the wall.
- Reach your arms out to the side, making a T, with your palms facing out (not toward the wall).
- Slowly, keeping the backs of the hands and wrists against the wall, work your arms overhead, stopping once the arms or the ribs pull away from the wall.
- Repeat in a smooth fashion, like you're making snow angels on the wall.

## SEATED & STANDING PIRIFORMIS STRETCH

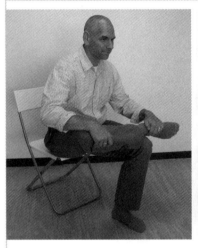 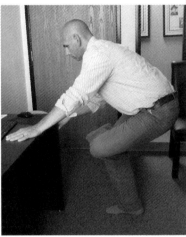

- Sitting on the edge of the chair, keep your left foot on the floor and cross your right leg over so the ankle is resting on the left knee.
- Untuck your pelvis—follow the protocol outlined for better sitting on page 38—and then slowly lean forward.
- For an additional challenge, do this stretch while standing. Using your desk for balance, hook the ankle of one leg over the knee of the other, then lower your hips toward the ground while keeping your standing leg's knee directly above the ankle.

## PELVIC SLIDE

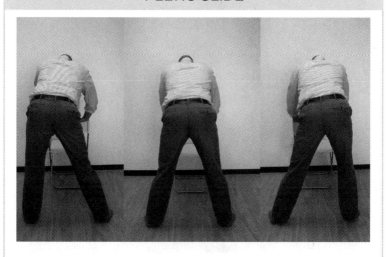

- Stand with your legs more than hip-width apart, feet pointing forward, with a chair or desk in front of you.
- Bend forward until your hands are resting on the seat of the chair, and relax your pelvis and spine toward the ground.
- Back up your hips until they are behind your heels (you'll feel your hamstrings start to stretch), and then shift your pelvis toward the right leg and then toward the left, without migrating forward.
- Don't allow your pelvis to migrate forward; the only motion should be a side-to-side gliding over the tops of the thighs.
- Changing the width of your feet will change the stretch.

## NERVE STRETCH

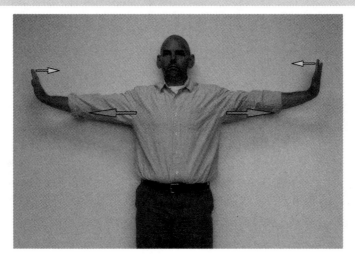

• Reach your hands away from you, making a T and a " STOP! In the name of love" motion with each hand.

• Spreading the fingers away from each other, slowly work your fingertips back toward the main axis of your body.

•  Keep your middle fingers pointing up, your thumbs pointing forward, and your elbow pits facing the ceiling.

• Think of reaching the entire arm bone away from you.

## THE WAITER

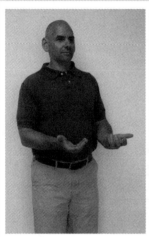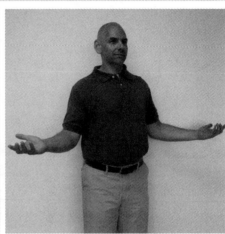

- Standing, bend your elbows to 90°, with your palms up like you're holding a tray in your hands.
- Keeping your hands up and your elbows bent, slowly move your hands laterally until your right hand is off to the right and your left to the left. Bring them back together.
- Initially you can do this *sans* equipment, but for even more work, do this motion using light-resistance exercise tubing or a set of hand weights (no more than five pounds).

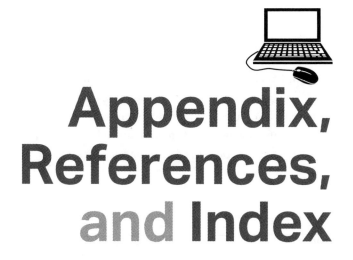

# Appendix,
# References,
# and Index

The following is a product guide designed to help cut down your search time (i.e. get you off of your computer faster) for some of the products I've mentioned or alluded to in this book. I have not tried all of these items personally, and this list isn't an endorsement; these are just products that seem to be in line with the goal of changing your body's geometry throughout the day and can be thought of as components to a dynamic workstation.

## FEET

*Note that I have very long lists of minimal shoe companies on my blog—just search there for shoes and you'll find lists of winter, summer, and children's shoes. Here are some other shoe and related resources:*

Fit in Clouds Shoes

Gaiam Restore Hot & Cold Foot Roller

Happy Feet Original Foot Alignment Socks

Kalso Earth Shoe

Merrell Barefoot Shoes

Planet Shoes

The Primal Professional Oxfords

Unshoes

Vibram Five Fingers

Xero Shoes

## KEYBOARDS

DataCal Ezsee Low Vision Keyboard Large Print Yellow Keys

ErgoTravel Keyboard

Goldtouch ErgoSecure 2.0 Smart Card Keyboard

Goldtouch V2 Adjustable Comfort Keyboard (for Mac and PC)

Herman Miller Keyboard Supports

Human Scale Build Your Own Keyboard

Kinesis Advantage Contoured Keyboard

Kinesis Advantage Pro Contoured USB Keyboard

Logitech K811 keyboard

Truly Ergonomic Keyboard Soft Tactile Model 207

## LIGHTING

ErgoMart FL18G lamp

Herman Miller Flute Personal Light

Herman Miller Tone Personal Light

Herman Miller Twist LED Task Light

Human Scale Diffrient Task Light

Human Scale Element Classic & 790

Human Scale Element Disc LED Light

Koncept Equo LED Task Lamp

Koncept LED Z Bar Task Light

Koncept Mosso LED Task Lamp

Philips L Prize Light Bulb

## MATS

Allegro Medical Cobblestone Mat

Barefoot Mats

Ergomat

Ergomat Infinity Bubble Mat

Ergomat Super Safe Mat

Gel Pro Ergo Comfort Rug

Gel Pro New Life Eco Pro

Global Industrial

New Pig

The Human Solution

The StreamBed Foot Reflexology Walking Mat

Topo mat by Ergodriven

## MICE

Aerobic Mouse

ErgoContour Mouse

Ergoguys Wow Pen Joy Optical Mouse

Evoluent Vertical Mouse Wireless

Goldtouch Bluetooth Comfort Mouse—Right Handed

Goldtouch Comfort Mouse—Left Handed

Goldtouch Wireless Ambidextrous Mouse

Handshoe Mouse Light Click Wireless

Mousetrapper Flexible Mouse

OrthoMouse

Penguin Vertical Mouse

## SOFTWARE

F.lux

Time Out Free

## STOOLS

ergoCentric Sit Stand II Standing Stool

Focal Upright Furniture Locus Leaning Seat

Focal Upright Furniture Mobis Leaning Stool

Focal Upright Furniture Mogo Portable Seat

Global Kneeling Chair

Herman Miller Bombo Stool

Herman Miller Lyra Stool

Herman Miller She Said Stool

Herman Miller Stool One

Humanscale Saddle/Pony Saddle seat

Knoll Jamaica Stool

Muvman Sit-Stand Stool

Office Master WS15 Sit to Stand Work Stool

Swopper Chair—Design Your Own

Swopper Muvman

Swopper Classic Stool

Uncaged Wobble Stool

Varier Move Standing Stool

Varier Multi Balans Kneeling Chair

Wigli Stool

## WORKSTATIONS

Anthro Technology Furniture

Chairigami Cardboard Standing Desk

ErgoDriven Standing Desk Calculator

Ergohuman

Ergotron

Focal Upright Furniture Workstations

Ninja Standing Desk

Stand in Good Health

The Standesk 2200

TreadDesk

Vari Desk

Zen Office WorkStation

## MISCELLANEOUS

Contour Lumbar Cushion

ContourSit Car Cushion

Dr. Cohen's Heatable AcuBack Kit

Ergonomic Accessories

FitBALL Seating Disk

Gaiam Restore Hot and Cold Therapy Kit

Gokhale Cushion

Squatty Potty

Yoga Tune Up Therapy Balls

Zen Office Eco Backrest

# references & additional reading

The most up-to-date literature on the health effects of sitting can be found at ncbi.nlm.nih.gov/pubmed or scholar.google.com.

You can use the following search terms:

"sitting time"

"time spent sitting"

"sedentarism"

"screen time sedentary"

"standing workstation"

Al-Dirini, R.M.A., Reed, M.P., & Thewlis, D. (2015). Deformation of the Gluteal Soft Tissues During Sitting. *Clinical Biomechanics.* Retrieved online: clinbiomech.com/article/S0268-0033(15)00144-8/abstract

American College of Cardiology. (2015). "Excess sitting linked to coronary artery calcification, an early indicator of heart problems." ScienceDaily, 5 March. Retrieved online: sciencedaily.com/releases/2015/03/150305205959.htm

Beers, E.A., Roemmich, J.N., Epstein, L.H., et al. (2008). Increasing Passive Energy Expenditure During Clerical Work. *European Journal of Applied Physiology, 103 (3),* 353-360.

Biswas, A., Oh, P.I., Faulkner, G.E., Bajaj, R.R., Silver, M.A., Mitchell, M.S., & Alter, D.A. (2015). Sedentary Time and Its Association for Risk With Disease Incidence, Mortality, and Hospitalization In Adults: A Systematic Review and Meta-Analysis. *Annals of Internal Medicine, 162 (2),* 123-132.

Chepesiuk, R. (2009). Missing The Dark: Health Effects of Light Pollution. *Environmental Health Perspectives, 117 (1),* A20-A27.

Crotty, T.P. (1991). The roles of turbulence and vasa vasorum in the aetiology of varicose veins. *Medical Hypotheses, 34(1),* 41-8.

Dosemeci, M., Hayes, R., Vetter, R., & Blair, A. (1993). Occupational physical activity, socioeconomic status, and risks of 15 cancer sites in Turkey. *Cancer Causes and Control, 4(4),* 313-321.

Dunstan, D., Barr, E., Healy, G., & Owen, N. (2010). Television Viewing Time and Mortality: the Australian Diabetes, Obesity and Lifestyle Study (AusDiab). *Circulation, 121,* 384-391.

Elsharawy, M., Naim, M., Abdelmaguid, E.M., Al-Mulhim, A. (2007). Role of saphenous vein wall in the pathogenesis of primary varicose veins. *Oxford Journal of Interactive CardioVascular and Thoracic Surgery, 6(2),* 219-224.

Hahn, C., & Schwartz, M.A. (2009). Mechanotransduction in Vascular Physiology and Atherogenesis. *Nature Reviews Molecular Cell Biology, 10,* 53-62.

Hall, J., Mansfield, L., Kay, T., & McConnell, A.K. (2015). The Effect of a Sit-Stand Workstation Intervention on Daily Sitting, Standing and Physical Activity: Protocol for a 12-Month Workplace Randomized Control Trial. *Bio Med Central Public Health, 15,* 152.

Hansraj, K.K. (2014). Assessment of Stresses in the Cervical Spine Caused by Posture and the Position of the Head. *Surgical Technology International, 25,* 277-279.

Hsieh, H-J, Liu, C-A, Huang, B., Tseng, A.H.H., & Wang, D. L. (2014). Shear-Induced Endothelial Mechanotransduction: The Interplay Between Reactive Oxygen Species (ROS) and Nitric Oxide (NO) and the Pathophysiological Implications. *Journal of Biomedical Science, 21,* 3.

Katzmarzyk, P., Church, T., Craig, C., & Bouchard, C. (2009). Sitting time and mortality from all causes, cardiovascular disease, and cancer. *Medicine & Science in Sports & Exercise, 41(5),* 998-1005.

Kitchel, E. (2000). The Effects of Blue Light on Ocular Health. *Journal of Visual Impairment & Blindness, 94(6),* 399.

Labonté-LeMoyne, É.,Santhanam, R., Léger, P., Courtemanche, F., Fredette, M., Sénécal, S. (2015). The Delayed Effect of Treadmill Desk Usage On Recall and Attention. *Computers in Human Behavior 46,* 1-5.

Levine, J.A. & Miller, J.M. (2007). The Energy Expenditure of Using a "Walk-and-Work" Desk for Office Workers With Obesity. *British Journal of Sports Medicine, 41 (9),* 558-61.

Li, F., Fisher, K. J., & Harmer, P. (2005). Improving physical function and blood pressure in older adults through cobblestone mat walking: a randomized trial. *Journal of the American Geriatrics Society, 53(8),* 1305-12.

Matthews, C.E., George, S.M., Moore, S.C., Bowles, H.R., Blair, A., Park, Y., Troiano, R.P., Hollenbeck, A., Schatzkin, A. (2012). Amount of time spent in sedentary behaviors and cause-specific mortality in US adults. *American Journal of Clinical Nutrition, 95(2)*, 437-45.

Müller-Bühl, U., Leutgeb, R., Engeser, P., Achankang, E.N., Szecsenyi, J., & Laux, G. (2012). Varicose Veins Are A Risk Factor For Deep Venous Thrombosis In General Practice Patients. *Vasa, 41(5)*, 360-365.

National Institute for Occupational Safety and Health. (1999). *Stress At Work*. NIOSH Publication number 99-101. Retrieved from Centers for Disease Control and Prevention (CDC) website, cdc.gov/niosh/docs/99-101/.

O'Brien, J.A., Edwards, H.E., Finlayson, K., & Kerr, G. (2012). Understanding the relationships between the calf muscle pump, ankle range of motion and healing for adults with venous leg ulcers: a review of the literature. *Wound Practice and Research, 20(2)*, 80-85.

Oppezzo, M., & Schwartz, D.L. (2014). Give Your Ideas Some Legs: The Positive Effect of Walking On Creative Thinking. *Journal of Experimental Psychology: Learning, Memory and Cognition, 40(4)* 1142-1152.

Owen, N., Bauman, A., Brown, W. (2009). Too much sitting: a novel and important predictor of chronic disease risk. *British Journal of Sports Medicine 43(2)*, 81-83.

Patel, A.V., Bernstein, L., Deka, A., Spencer Feigelson, H., Campbell, P.T., Gapstur, S. M., Colditz, G.A., & Thun, M.J. (2010). Leisure Time Spent Sitting in Relation to Total Mortality in a Prospective Cohort of US Adults. *American Journal of Epidemiology, 172(4)*, 419-429.

Qiao, T., Liu, C., & Ran, F. (2005). The Impact of Gastrocnemius Muscle Cell Changes in Chronic Venous Insufficiency. *European Journal of Vascular and Endovascular Surgery, 30(4)*, 430-436.

Salmon, M. (2003). Artificial night lighting and sea turtles. *Biologist, 50(4)*, 163-168.

Shoham, N., Gottlieb, R., Shaharabani-Yosef, O., Zaretsky, U., Benayahu, D., Gefen, A. (2011). Static Mechanical Stretching Accelerates Lipid Production in 3T3-L1 Adipocytes by Activating the MEK Signaling Pathway. *American Journal of Physiology - Cell Physiology*, October, C429-C441.

Stamatakis, E., Hamer, M., & Dunstan, D. (2011). Screen-based entertainment time, all-cause mortality, and cardiovascular events: Population-based study with ongoing mortality and hospital events follow-up. *Journal of the American College of Cardiology, 18(57)*, 292-9.

Stvrtinová, V., Kolesár, J., & Wimmer, G. (1991). Prevalence of varicose veins of the lower limbs in the women working at a department store. *International Angiology: a Journal of the International Union of Angiology, 10(1)*, 2-5.

Takase, S., Pascarella, L., Bergan, J., & Schmid-Schonbein, G.W. (2004). Hypertension-induced venous valve remodeling. *Journal of Vascular Surgery, 39(6)*, 1329-34.

Thosar, S.S., Bielko, S.L., Mather, K.J., Johnston, J.D., & Wallace, J.P. (2015). Effect of Prolonged Sitting and Breaks in Sitting Time on Endothelial Function. *Medicine and Science in Sports and Exercise, 47(4)*, 843-849.

Töchsen, F., Krause, N., Hannerz, H., Burr, H., & Kristensen, T.S. (2000). Standing at work and varicose veins. *Scandinavian Journal of Work and Environmental Health, 26(5)*, 414-20.

Tudor-Locke, C., Schuna, J.M. Jr., Frensham, L.J., & Proenca, M. (2014). Changing The Way We Work: Elevating Energy Expenditure With Workstation Alternatives. *International Journal of Obesity, 38(6)*, 755-765.

Turner, C. (1998). Three rules for bone adaptation to mechanical stimuli. *Bone, 23(5)*, 399-407.

Tzima, E., Irani-Tehrani, M., Kiosses, W.B., Dejana, E., Schultz, D.A., Englehardt, B., Cao, G., DeLisser, H., & Schwartz, M.A. (2005). A Mechanosensory Complex that Mediates the Endothelial Cell Response to Fluid Shear Stress. *Nature, 437*, 426-431.

Whitfield, G., Pettee Gabriel, K., & Kohl, H. (2014). Sedentary and active: self-reported sitting time among marathon and half-marathon participants. *Journal of Physical Activity and Health, 11(1)*, 165-72.

# index

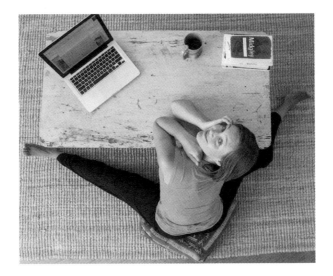

A biomechanist by training and a problem-solver at heart, Katy Bowman has the ability to blend a scientific approach with straight talk about sensible solutions and an unwavering sense of humor, earning her legions of followers. Her award-winning blog and podcast, *Katy Says*, reach hundreds of thousands of people every month, and thousands have taken her live classes. Her books, the bestselling *Move Your DNA* (2014*), Every Woman's Guide to Foot Pain Relief: The New Science of Healthy Feet* (2011), *Alignment Matters* (2013), and *Whole Body Barefoot* (2015), have been critically acclaimed and translated worldwide. In between her book writing efforts, Katy travels the globe to teach Nutritious Movement™ courses in person, and spends as much time as possible moving outside with her husband and two young children.